BLACKWELL'S
UNDERGROUND CLINICAL VIGNETTES

PHARMACOLOGY, 3E

BLACKWELL'S
UNDERGROUND CLINICAL VIGNETTES

PHARMACOLOGY, 3E

VIKAS BHUSHAN, MD
University of California, San Francisco, Class of 1991
Series Editor, Diagnostic Radiologist

VISHAL PALL, MBBS
Government Medical College, Chandigarh, India, Class of 1996
Series Editor, U. of Texas, Galveston, Resident in Internal Medicine &
Preventive Medicine

TAO LE, MD
University of California, San Francisco, Class of 1996

HOANG NGUYEN, MD, MBA
Northwestern University, Class of 2001

CONTRIBUTORS

Abby Geltemeyer, MD
University of Texas, Houston, Resident in Medicine/Pediatrics

Jose M. Fierro, MD
La Salle University, Mexico City

Mae Sheikh-Ali, MD
University of Damascus, Syria, Class of 1999

Kris Alden
University of Illinois – Chicago, Medical Scientist Training Program

Vipal Soni, MD
UCLA School of Medicine, Class of 1999

FACULTY REVIEWER

Bertram Katzung, MD, PHD
Professor Emeritus of Pharmacology, UCSF School of Medicine

© 2002 by Blackwell Science, Inc.

Editorial Offices:

Commerce Place, 350 Main Street, Malden,
    Massachusetts 02148, USA
Osney Mead, Oxford OX2 0EL, England
25 John Street, London WC1N 2BS, England
23 Ainslie Place, Edinburgh EH3 6AJ, Scotland
54 University Street, Carlton, Victoria 3053,
    Australia

Other Editorial Offices:

Blackwell Wissenschafts-Verlag GmbH,
    Kurfürstendamm 57, 10707 Berlin, Germany
Blackwell Science KK, MG Kodenmacho Building,
    7-10 Kodenmacho Nihombashi, Chuo-ku,
    Tokyo 104, Japan
Iowa State University Press, A Blackwell Science
    Company, 2121 S. State Avenue, Ames, Iowa
    50014-8300, USA

Acquisitions: Laura DeYoung
Development: Amy Nuttbrock
Production: Lorna Hind and Shawn Girsberger
Manufacturing: Lisa Flanagan
Marketing Manager: Kathleen Mulcahy
Cover design by Leslie Haimes
Interior design by Shawn Girsberger
Typeset by TechBooks
Printed and bound by Capital City Press

Blackwell's Underground Clinical Vignettes:
    Pharmacology, 3e
ISBN 0-632-04557-4

Printed in the United States of America
02 03 04 05 5 4 3 2 1

First Indian Reprint 2002

Printed and bound by Multivista Global Limited,
Chennai - 600 042.

The Blackwell Science logo is a trade mark of
Blackwell Science Ltd., registered at the United
Kingdom Trade Marks Registry

Library of Congress Cataloging-in-Publication Data
Bhushan, Vikas.
Blackwell's underground clinical vignettes.
Pharmacology / author, Vikas Bhushan. – 3rd ed.
    p. ; cm. – (Underground clinical vignettes)
Rev. ed. of: Pharmacology / Vikas Bhushan ... [et al.].
c1999. ISBN 0-632-04557-4 (pbk.)
1. Pharmacology – Case studies. 2. Physicians –
Licenses – United States – Examinations –
Study guides.
    [DNLM: 1. Pharmacology – Case Report.
2. Pharmacology – Problems and Exercises. QV 18.2
B575b 2002] I. Title: Underground clinical vignettes.
Pharmacology. II. Title: Pharmacology.
III. Pharmacology. IV. Title. V. Series.
    RM301 .B465 2002
    615'.1'076–dc21

                                        2001004930

Notice

The authors of this volume have taken care that the information contained herein is accurate and compatible with the standards generally accepted at the time of publication. Nevertheless, it is difficult to ensure that all the information given is entirely accurate for all circumstances. The publisher and authors do not guarantee the contents of this book and disclaim any liability, loss, or damage incurred as a consequence, directly or indirectly, of the use and application of any of the contents of this volume.

CONTENTS

ACKNOWLEDGMENTS

Throughout the production of this book, we have had the support of many friends and colleagues. Special thanks to our support team including Anu Gupta, Andrea Fellows, Anastasia Anderson, Srishti Gupta, Mona Pall, Jonathan Kirsch and Chirag Amin. For prior contributions we thank Gianni Le Nguyen, Tarun Mathur, Alex Grimm, Sonia Santos and Elizabeth Sanders.

We have enjoyed working with a world-class international publishing group at Blackwell Science, including Laura DeYoung, Amy Nuttbrock, Lisa Flanagan, Shawn Girsberger, Lorna Hind and Gordon Tibbitts. For help with securing images for the entire series we also thank Lee Martin, Kristopher Jones, Tina Panizzi and Peter Anderson at the University of Alabama, the Armed Forces Institute of Pathology, and many of our fellow Blackwell Science authors.

For submitting comments, corrections, editing, proofreading, and assistance across all of the vignette titles in all editions, we collectively thank:

Tara Adamovich, Carolyn Alexander, Kris Alden, Henry E. Aryan, Lynman Bacolor, Natalie Barteneva, Dean Bartholomew, Debashish Behera, Sumit Bhatia, Sanjay Bindra, Dave Brinton, Julianne Brown, Alexander Brownie, Tamara Callahan, David Canes, Bryan Casey, Aaron Caughey, Hebert Chen, Jonathan Cheng, Arnold Cheung, Arnold Chin, Simion Chiosea, Yoon Cho, Samuel Chung, Gretchen Conant, Vladimir Coric, Christopher Cosgrove, Ronald Cowan, Karekin R. Cunningham, A. Sean Dalley, Rama Dandamudi, Sunit Das, Ryan Armando Dave, John David, Emmanuel de la Cruz, Robert DeMello, Navneet Dhillon, Sharmila Dissanaike, David Donson, Adolf Etchegaray, Alea Eusebio, Priscilla A. Frase, David Frenz, Kristin Gaumer, Yohannes Gebreegziabher, Anil Gehi, Tony George, L.M. Gotanco, Parul Goyal, Alex Grimm, Rajeev Gupta, Ahmad Halim, Sue Hall, David Hasselbacher, Tamra Heimert, Michelle Higley, Dan Hoit, Eric Jackson, Tim Jackson, Sundar Jayaraman, Pei-Ni Jone, Aarchan Joshi, Rajni K. Jutla, Faiyaz Kapadi, Seth Karp, Aaron S. Kesselheim, Sana Khan, Andrew Pin-wei Ko, Francis Kong, Paul Konitzky, Warren S. Krackov, Benjamin H.S. Lau, Ann LaCasce, Connie Lee, Scott Lee, Guillermo Lehmann, Kevin Leung, Paul Levett, Warren Levinson, Eric Ley, Ken Lin,

Pavel Lobanov, J. Mark Maddox, Aram Mardian, Samir Mehta, Gil Melmed, Joe Messina, Robert Mosca, Michael Murphy, Vivek Nandkarni, Siva Naraynan, Carvell Nguyen, Linh Nguyen, Deanna Nobleza, Craig Nodurft, George Noumi, Darin T. Okuda, Adam L. Palance, Paul Pamphrus, Jinha Park, Sonny Patel, Ricardo Pietrobon, Riva L. Rahl, Aashita Randeria, Rachan Reddy, Beatriu Reig, Marilou Reyes, Jeremy Richmon, Tai Roe, Rick Roller, Rajiv Roy, Diego Ruiz, Anthony Russell, Sanjay Sahgal, Urmimala Sarkar, John Schilling, Isabell Schmitt, Daren Schuhmacher, Sonal Shah, Fadi Abu Shahin, Mae Sheikh-Ali, Edie Shen, Justin Smith, John Stulak, Lillian Su, Julie Sundaram, Rita Suri, Seth Sweetser, Antonio Talayero, Merita Tan, Mark Tanaka, Eric Taylor, Jess Thompson, Indi Trehan, Raymond Turner, Okafo Uchenna, Eric Uyguanco, Richa Varma, John Wages, Alan Wang, Eunice Wang, Andy Weiss, Amy Williams, Brian Yang, Hany Zaky, Ashraf Zaman and David Zipf.

For generously contributing images to the entire *Underground Clinical Vignette* Step 1 series, we collectively thank the staff at Blackwell Science in Oxford, Boston, and Berlin as well as:

- Axford, J. *Medicine.* Osney Mead: Blackwell Science Ltd, 1996. Figures 2.14, 2.15, 2.16, 2.27, 2.28, 2.31, 2.35, 2.36, 2.38, 2.43, 2.65a, 2.65b, 2.65c, 2.103b, 2.105b, 3.20b, 3.21, 8.27, 8.27b, 8.77b, 8.77c, 10.81b, 10.96a, 12.28a, 14.6, 14.16, 14.50.

- Bannister B, Begg N, Gillespie S. *Infectious Disease, 2nd Edition.* Osney Mead: Blackwell Science Ltd, 2000. Figures 2.8, 3.4, 5.28, 18.10, W5.32, W5.6.

- Berg D. *Advanced Clinical Skills and Physical Diagnosis.* Blackwell Science Ltd., 1999. Figures 7.10, 7.12, 7.13, 7.2, 7.3, 7.7, 7.8, 7.9, 8.1, 8.2, 8.4, 8.5, 9.2, 10.2, 11.3, 11.5, 12.6.

- Cuschieri A, Hennessy TPJ, Greenhalgh RM, Rowley DA, Grace PA. *Clinical Surgery.* Osney Mead: Blackwell Science Ltd, 1996. Figures 13.19, 18.22, 18.33.

- Gillespie SH, Bamford K. *Medical Microbiology and Infection at a Glance.* Osney Mead: Blackwell Science Ltd, 2000. Figures 20, 23.

- Ginsberg L. *Lecture Notes on Neurology, 7th Edition.* Osney Mead: Blackwell Science Ltd, 1999. Figures 12.3, 18.3, 18.3b.

- Elliott T, Hastings M, Desselberger U. *Lecture Notes on Medical Microbiology, 3rd Edition.* Osney Mead: Blackwell Science Ltd, 1997. Figures 2, 5, 7, 8, 9, 11, 12, 14, 15, 16, 17, 19, 20, 25, 26, 27, 29, 30, 34, 35, 52.

- Mehta AB, Hoffbrand AV. *Haematology at a Glance*. Osney Mead: Blackwell Science Ltd, 2000. Figures 22.1, 22.2, 22.3.

Please let us know if your name has been missed or misspelled and we will be happy to make the update in the next edition.

PREFACE TO THE 3RD EDITION

We were very pleased with the overwhelmingly positive student feedback for the 2nd edition of our *Underground Clinical Vignettes* series. Well over 100,000 copies of the UCV books are in print and have been used by students all over the world.

Over the last two years we have accumulated and incorporated **over a thousand "updates"** and improvements suggested by you, our readers, including:

- many additions of specific boards and wards testable content

- deletions of redundant and overlapping cases

- reordering and reorganization of all cases in both series

- a new master index by case name in each Atlas

- correction of a few factual errors

- diagnosis and treatment updates

- addition of 5–20 new cases in every book

- and the addition of clinical exam photographs within *UCV— Anatomy.*

And most important of all, the third edition sets now include two brand new **COLOR ATLAS** supplements, one for each Clinical Vignette series.

- The *UCV–Basic Science Color Atlas* (*Step 1*) includes over 250 color plates, divided into gross pathology, microscopic pathology (histology), hematology, and microbiology (smears).

- The *UCV–Clinical Science Color Atlas* (*Step 2*) has over 125 color plates, including patient images, dermatology, and funduscopy.

Each atlas image is descriptively captioned and linked to its corresponding Step 1 case, Step 2 case, and/or Step 2 MiniCase.

How Atlas Links Work:

Step 1 Book Codes are:
A = Anatomy
BS = Behavioral Science
BC = Biochemistry
M1 = Microbiology, Vol. I
M2 = Microbiology, Vol. II
P1 = Pathophysiology, Vol. I
P2 = Pathophysiology, Vol. II
P3 = Pathophysiology, Vol. III
PH = Pharmacology

Step 2 Book Codes are:
ER = Emergency Medicine
IM1 = Internal Medicine, Vol. I
IM2 = Internal Medicine, Vol. II
NEU = Neurology
OB = OB/GYN
PED = Pediatrics
SUR = Surgery
PSY = Psychiatry
MC = MiniCase

Case Number

UCV1 M-P3-032A   UCV2 ER-035A, ER-035B

Indicates Type of Image: H = Hematology
M = Microbiology
PG = Gross Pathology
PM = Microscopic Pathology

Indicates UCV1 or UCV2 Series

- If the Case number (032, 035, etc.) is not followed by a letter, then there is only one image. Otherwise A, B, C, D indicate up to 4 images.

Bold Faced Links: In order to give you access to the largest number of images possible, we have chosen to cross link the Step 1 and 2 series.

- If the link is bold-faced this indicates that the link is direct (i.e., Step 1 Case with the Basic Science Step 1 Atlas link).
- If the link is not bold-faced this indicates that the link is indirect (Step 1 case with Clinical Science Step 2 Atlas link or vice versa).

We have also implemented a few structural changes upon your request:

- Each current and future edition of our popular *First Aid for the USMLE Step 1* (Appleton & Lange/McGraw-Hill) and *First Aid for the USMLE Step 2* (Appleton & Lange/McGraw-Hill) book will be linked to the corresponding UCV case.
- We eliminated UCV → First Aid links as they frequently become out of date, as the *First Aid* books are revised yearly.

- The Color Atlas is also specially designed for quizzing—captions are descriptive and do not give away the case name directly.

We hope the updated UCV series will remain a unique and well-integrated study tool that provides compact clinical correlations to basic science information. They are designed to be easy and fun (comparatively) to read, and helpful for both licensing exams and the wards.

We invite your corrections and suggestions for the fourth edition of these books. For the first submission of each factual correction or new vignette that is selected for inclusion in the fourth edition, you will receive a personal acknowledgment in the revised book. If you submit over 20 high-quality corrections, additions or new vignettes we will also consider **inviting you to become a "Contributor" on the book of your choice**. If you are interested in becoming a potential "Contributor" or "Author" on a future UCV book, or working with our team in developing additional books, please also e-mail us your CV/resume.

We prefer that you submit corrections or suggestions via electronic mail to **UCVteam@yahoo.com**. Please include "Underground Vignettes" as the subject of your message. If you do not have access to e-mail, use the following mailing address: Blackwell Publishing, Attn: UCV Editors, 350 Main Street, Malden, MA 02148, USA.

Vikas Bhushan
Vishal Pall
Tao Le
October 2001

HOW TO USE THIS BOOK

This series was originally developed to address the increasing number of clinical vignette questions on medical examinations, including the USMLE Step 1 and Step 2. It is also designed to supplement and complement the popular *First Aid for the USMLE Step 1* (Appleton & Lange/McGraw Hill) and *First Aid for the USMLE Step 2* (Appleton & Lange/McGraw Hill).

Each UCV 1 book uses a series of approximately 100 **"supra-prototypical" cases as a way to condense testable facts and associations**. The clinical vignettes in this series are designed to incorporate as many testable facts as possible into a cohesive and memorable clinical picture. The vignettes represent composites drawn from general and specialty textbooks, reference books, thousands of USMLE style questions and the personal experience of the authors and reviewers.

Although each case tends to present all the signs, symptoms, and diagnostic findings for a particular illness, **patients generally will not present with such a "complete" picture either clinically or on a medical examination**. Cases are not meant to simulate a potential real patient or an exam vignette. All the **boldfaced "buzzwords" are for learning purposes** and are not necessarily expected to be found in any one patient with the disease.

Definitions of selected important terms are placed within the vignettes in (SMALL CAPS) in parentheses. Other parenthetical remarks often refer to the pathophysiology or mechanism of disease. The format should also help students learn to present cases succinctly during oral "bullet" presentations on clinical rotations. The cases are meant to serve as a condensed review, not as a primary reference. The information provided in this book has been prepared with a great deal of thought and careful research. This book should not, however, be considered as your sole source of information. Corrections, suggestions and submissions of new cases are encouraged and will be acknowledged and incorporated when appropriate in future editions.

ABBREVIATIONS

5-ASA	5-aminosalicylic acid
ABGs	arterial blood gases
ABVD	adriamycin/bleomycin/vincristine/dacarbazine
ACE	angiotensin-converting enzyme
ACTH	adrenocorticotropic hormone
ADH	antidiuretic hormone
AFP	alpha fetal protein
AI	aortic insufficiency
AIDS	acquired immunodeficiency syndrome
ALL	acute lymphocytic leukemia
ALT	alanine transaminase
AML	acute myelogenous leukemia
ANA	antinuclear antibody
ARDS	adult respiratory distress syndrome
ASD	atrial septal defect
ASO	anti-streptolysin O
AST	aspartate transaminase
AV	arteriovenous
BE	barium enema
BP	blood pressure
BUN	blood urea nitrogen
CAD	coronary artery disease
CALLA	common acute lymphoblastic leukemia antigen
CBC	complete blood count
CHF	congestive heart failure
CK	creatine kinase
CLL	chronic lymphocytic leukemia
CML	chronic myelogenous leukemia
CMV	cytomegalovirus
CNS	central nervous system
COPD	chronic obstructive pulmonary disease
CPK	creatine phosphokinase
CSF	cerebrospinal fluid
CT	computed tomography
CVA	cerebrovascular accident
CXR	chest x-ray
DIC	disseminated intravascular coagulation
DIP	distal interphalangeal
DKA	diabetic ketoacidosis
DM	diabetes mellitus
DTRs	deep tendon reflexes
DVT	deep venous thrombosis

EBV	Epstein–Barr virus
ECG	electrocardiography
Echo	echocardiography
EF	ejection fraction
EGD	esophagogastroduodenoscopy
EMG	electromyography
ERCP	endoscopic retrograde cholangiopancreatography
ESR	erythrocyte sedimentation rate
FEV	forced expiratory volume
FNA	fine needle aspiration
FTA-ABS	fluorescent treponemal antibody absorption
FVC	forced vital capacity
GFR	glomerular filtration rate
GH	growth hormone
GI	gastrointestinal
GM-CSF	granulocyte macrophage colony stimulating factor
GU	genitourinary
HAV	hepatitis A virus
hcG	human chorionic gonadotrophin
HEENT	head, eyes, ears, nose, and throat
HIV	human immunodeficiency virus
HLA	human leukocyte antigen
HPI	history of present illness
HR	heart rate
HRIG	human rabies immune globulin
HS	hereditary spherocytosis
ID/CC	identification and chief complaint
IDDM	insulin-dependent diabetes mellitus
Ig	immunoglobulin
IGF	insulin-like growth factor
IM	intramuscular
JVP	jugular venous pressure
KUB	kidneys/ureter/bladder
LDH	lactate dehydrogenase
LES	lower esophageal sphincter
LFTs	liver function tests
LP	lumbar puncture
LV	left ventricular
LVH	left ventricular hypertrophy
Lytes	electrolytes
MCHC	mean corpuscular hemoglobin concentration
MCV	mean corpuscular volume
MEN	multiple endocrine neoplasia

MGUS	monoclonal gammopathy of undetermined significance
MHC	major histocompatibility complex
MI	myocardial infarction
MOPP	mechlorethamine/vincristine (Oncovorin)/ procarbazine/prednisone
MR	magnetic resonance (imaging)
NHL	non-Hodgkin's lymphoma
NIDDM	non-insulin-dependent diabetes mellitus
NPO	nil per os (nothing by mouth)
NSAID	nonsteroidal anti-inflammatory drug
PA	posteroanterior
PIP	proximal interphalangeal
PBS	peripheral blood smear
PE	physical exam
PFTs	pulmonary function tests
PMI	point of maximal intensity
PMN	polymorphonuclear leukocyte
PT	prothrombin time
PTCA	percutaneous transluminal angioplasty
PTH	parathyroid hormone
PTT	partial thromboplastin time
PUD	peptic ulcer disease
RBC	red blood cell
RPR	rapid plasma reagin
RR	respiratory rate
RS	Reed–Sternberg (cell)
RV	right ventricular
RVH	right ventricular hypertrophy
SBFT	small bowel follow-through
SIADH	syndrome of inappropriate secretion of ADH
SLE	systemic lupus erythematosus
STD	sexually transmitted disease
TFTs	thyroid function tests
tPA	tissue plasminogen activator
TSH	thyroid-stimulating hormone
TIBC	total iron-binding capacity
TIPS	transjugular intrahepatic portosystemic shunt
TPO	thyroid peroxidase
TSH	thyroid-stimulating hormone
TTP	thrombotic thrombocytopenic purpura
UA	urinalysis
UGI	upper GI
US	ultrasound

VDRL	Venereal Disease Research Laboratory
VS	vital signs
VT	ventricular tachycardia
WBC	white blood cell
WPW	Wolff–Parkinson–White (syndrome)
XR	x-ray

ID/CC A 45-year-old female who works as a preschool teacher complains of **fatigue**, headache, dizziness, dry cough, **shortness of breath**, and **constipation**.

HPI She has been receiving **amiodarone** for 1 year for treatment for chronic palpitations that arose spontaneously, with tachycardia that reaches 220 beats per minute (SUPRAVENTRICULAR TACHYCARDIA) and increases when she drinks coffee, is under stress, or smokes.

PE VS: **bradycardia** (HR 55); BP normal; no fever. PE: well hydrated, conscious, and oriented; no neck masses or bruit; **diffuse crackling sounds and wheezes** in both lung fields, predominantly in bases; abdominal and neurologic exams normal; violaceous skin discoloration in sun-exposed areas.

Labs ECG: **prolonged QT interval** and QRS duration. **AST and ALT moderately elevated**.

Imaging CXR: bilateral interstitial infiltrates (incipient pulmonary fibrosis).

Treatment Continuously monitor ECG and vital signs. Sodium bicarbonate may reverse cardiac depressant effects if evident. Discontinue drug if evidence of pulmonary fibrosis.

Discussion Amiodarone is a class IA and III antiarrhythmic drug. Adverse reactions require careful monitoring and include **thyroid dysfunction** (both hypo- and hyperthyroidism), **constipation, hepatocellular necrosis**, and **pulmonary fibrosis**, which may be fatal. It may also produce **bradycardia** and **heart block** in susceptible individuals. Amiodarone has a **long half-life**, so if toxicity occurs, it persists long after the drug has been discontinued. Amiodarone increases the blood levels of digoxin, phenytoin, and warfarin.

AMIODARONE SIDE EFFECTS

ID/CC   A 54-year-old obese male who is the owner of a chain of fast-food restaurants is brought to the ER after **fainting at work**; earlier in the morning he complained of **dizziness and dyspnea**.

HPI   He had been having episodes of acute, severe retrosternal chest pain associated with exercise or stress (ANGINA PECTORIS) for over 2 years and is taking **propranolol**.

PE   VS: **hypotension (BP 85/60); bradycardia** (HR 52); no fever. PE: patient is conscious; lung fields have **scattered wheezes** (BRONCHOSPASM); no hepatosplenomegaly or peritoneal signs.

Labs   ECG: QRS normal, but **P-R interval increased** (FIRST-DEGREE AV BLOCK).

Treatment   Treat bradycardia with atropine or epinephrine. Treat **bronchospasm** with bronchodilators. Treat hypotension with fluids and norepinephrine. Glucagon can be life-saving.

Discussion   Propranolol is a competitive nonselective beta-blocker that acts at both β_1 and β_2 receptors. β_2 receptors are found in bronchiolar and vascular smooth muscle. Uses include management of hypertension and tachyarrhythmias, hypertrophic cardiomyopathy, prevention of angina and migraines, reduction of mortality after myocardial infarction, and treatment of glaucoma and hyperthyroidism. Overdose can present with cardiac conduction disturbances, severe CNS toxicity (seizures, coma), and hyperkalemia.

ID/CC A 62-year-old female is referred to a pulmonary medicine specialist by her family physician because of a **chronic dry cough** that has been **unresponsive to medications**.

HPI On careful, directed questioning, the specialist discovers that she had been taking **captopril** for hypertension for 3 years. She also complains of **taste changes** and a **rash** on her chest and lower legs.

PE VS: normal. PE: no lymphadenopathy; funduscopic exam reveals grade I hypertensive retinopathy; discrete nonpruritic maculopapular **rash** on legs and chest.

Labs Serum **renin increased; angiotensin II decreased**. Lytes: hyperkalemia. CBC/PFTs: normal. LFTs: normal. UA: mild **proteinuria**.

Imaging CXR: no signs of COPD, neoplasm, or other pathology that would account for cough.

Treatment Aspirin, nifedipine, or cromolyn may decrease cough. However, it may be necessary to switch to another antihypertensive. **Losartan** is an alternative agent that blocks the binding of angiotensin II to its receptor and does not cause cough.

Discussion Captopril is an ACE inhibitor and thus reduces levels of angiotensin II and prevents the inactivation of bradykinin (a potent vasodilator). It is used to treat hypertension, CHF, and diabetic renal disease. It is **contraindicated in pregnancy** because of fetotoxicity; other side effects are **cough, hypotension, taste changes, rash, proteinuria, hyperkalemia, angioedema**, and **neutropenia**.

ID/CC   A 54-year-old white female complains of intermittent **nausea and vomiting, headaches, fatigue**, and **blurred vision** over the past 3 months.

HPI   She describes objects as **appearing yellow** to her. She has a history of heart failure with **chronic digoxin** use as well as **diuretics** (may induce hypokalemia).

PE   VS: **bradycardia** (HR 48); BP normal; no fever. PE: in no acute distress; slight increase in JVP; S3 present; rales at lung bases; mild hepatomegaly; ankle edema.

Labs   CBC: normal. Lytes: **hypokalemia**. Elevated BUN; elevated creatinine. ECG: **second-degree AV block with AV junctional rhythm**.

Imaging   CXR: moderate enlargement of the heart (due to long-standing CHF); no signs of lung infection.

Treatment   Lower and space apart the dose. Correct hypokalemia. Digoxin-specific Fab antibody fragments.

Discussion   Digoxin is a cardiac glycoside that inhibits the Na-K ATP-ase of cell membranes, causing an increase in intracellular sodium that results in an elevation in the intracellular calcium level, thereby causing positive inotropy. **Renal failure may precipitate toxicity** at normal therapeutic doses (excretion is decreased). Hypokalemia is a frequent predisposing factor for toxicity. ECG changes may vary widely; AV conduction disturbances, such as PAT with block, are characteristic, as are bigeminy, bradycardia, and flattened T waves.

ID/CC   An anesthesiologist is summoned into the OR when a 34-year-old male undergoing a **routine hernia repair** begins to have **seizures**.

HPI   The surgeon was chatting with the chief resident while injecting **lidocaine** subcutaneously for a local anesthetic repair when the patient suddenly started having slurred speech, tremors, and **tonic-clonic convulsions** (lidocaine was inadvertently injected systemically into the inferior epigastric vessels).

PE   Lips and fingertips blue (CYANOSIS); patient **biting his tongue**; eyes rolled inward; spastic extremities and spine with shaking movements during intervals.

Labs   There was no time to take blood samples.

Treatment   Control seizures with IV diazepam or barbiturates. Intubate, oxygenate, and ventilate in anticipation of second phase (respiratory depression).

Discussion   Lidocaine is an amide that blocks sodium channels, primarily in rapidly firing cells such as those in the myocardium, in pain fibers, and in the CNS. Overdosage occurs with inadvertent systemic injection, mainly in obstetric and surgical procedures, and is manifested by CNS toxicity (seizures) and a "hyper" state. This is **followed by a depressive period** with obtundation, hypotension, and **cardiorespiratory depression**. Toxicity should be differentiated from the infrequent anaphylactic reaction.

ID/CC A 52-year-old man visits his physician complaining of **extreme tiredness, dry mouth, and easy fatigability**; he states that he has never experienced symptoms such as these before.

HPI He was started on hydrochlorothiazide for treatment of hypertension, but it did not control his hypertension, so **α-methyldopa** was added approximately 2 months ago. On directed questioning, he states that he has been suffering from **sexual dysfunction** (impotence and inability to ejaculate) for the past several weeks.

PE VS: BP 130/90, but when standing up it is 100/60 (ORTHOSTATIC HYPOTENSION); no fever; bradycardia (HR 58). PE: **conjunctival pallor**; oriented with regard to person, time, and place; well hydrated despite **dryness of mouth**; funduscopic exam normal; no neck masses or bruits; no lymphadenopathy; chest auscultation normal; abdomen soft and nontender with no masses; no peritoneal signs.

Labs CBC: **positive Coombs' test**; decreased hemoglobin and hematocrit; **increased reticulocytes; decreased haptoglobin**. UA: hemoglobinuria. Increased indirect bilirubin; normal iron levels; **AST and ALT moderately increased**.

Imaging CXR/KUB: normal for age.

Treatment Switch antihypertensive treatment.

Discussion Methyldopa is a sympatholytic that produces a false neurotransmitter, α-methyl-norepinephrine, which activates inhibitory α2-receptors in the CNS. It is used as an antihypertensive drug, and its side effects include **impotence, Coombs positivity** (20% of patients), and, more rarely, **hemolytic anemia**. It can also cause **sedation, drowsiness**, severe orthostatic hypotension, and hepatic toxicity.

ID/CC The 48-year-old chief executive officer of a leading auto manufacturer is put on **niacin** and a restricted diet for the treatment of **high-LDL cholesterol**.

HPI The patient is a "bon vivant" who enjoys **drinking** and **eating** gourmet food as well as **smoking** two packs a day of Cuban filter-free dark tobacco cigarettes. On a visit two months afterward, the patient's lab tests show improvement, but he complains of **facial flushing** and **itching** on the lower back, palms, and anus.

PE VS: mild hypertension (BP 145/95). PE: obesity; **face, neck, and chest flushed**; no skin rash demonstrable on inspection.

Labs Serum glucose elevated (157 mg/dL); **LDL lowered** considerably in comparison to last visit; **triglycerides decreased**, but not as markedly; **HDL increased; AST and ALT** mildly **elevated; elevated uric acid; normal** levels of 5-hydroxyindoleacetic acid (vs. carcinoid syndrome, which may also produce facial flushing).

Imaging CXR: normal.

Treatment Flushing and itching are often transient. Aspirin diminishes symptoms by inhibiting prostaglandin synthesis.

Discussion Nicotinic acid (NIACIN) is a derivative of tryptophan, a constituent of NAD and NADP that is used in redox reactions. As a drug, it is used for its lipid-lowering properties (decreases VLDL, decreases LDL, and increases HDL cholesterol). **Hepatitis, hyperglycemia**, and exacerbation of peptic ulcer are other side effects.

ID/CC	A 53-year-old male **chemical-factory worker** presents with **chronic headaches and dizziness** with occasional **chest pain**.
HPI	The patient states that his headaches and dizziness occur most frequently when he **returns to work** after a few days off; he is otherwise in good health.
PE	VS: mild hypertension. PE: patient appears normal but **slightly cyanotic**; neck exam shows no masses or carotid bruit; cardiac exam normal; lung fields clear; abdomen soft and nontender; no hepatosplenomegaly; no focal neurologic signs.
Labs	CBC: normal. SMA-7 normal. UA: normal. **Methemoglobin levels elevated**. ECG: no sign of ischemia or necrosis.
Imaging	CXR/KUB: within normal limits for age.
Treatment	Hemodialysis and hemoperfusion are not effective in chronic nitrate exposure; monitor vital signs.
Discussion	Nitrates are a large class of drugs that are used in treatment of angina. All agents in this group, including nitroglycerin, act through nitric oxide (NO) release. NO, in turn, is a potent vasodilator of vascular smooth muscle. These compounds have a short half-life and may **produce tolerance in chronically exposed individuals**. Patients may suffer **angina or MI** as a result of **rebound coronary vasoconstriction** due to withdrawal.

ID/CC A 58-year-old man comes to see his cardiologist because of an **increased need for nitroglycerin patches** in order to control his oppressive exercise-induced chest pain (ANGINA).

HPI In the past, taking one tablet five minutes before physical activity controlled his symptoms; now he has to take two tablets. The patient has continued to smoke two packs of cigarettes each day and is concerned that his cardiac condition is worsening because of this **increased need for medication**.

PE VS: BP normal. PE: obese male in no acute distress; no rales or crackles on lung fields; heart sounds normal; no murmurs; no third or fourth heart sounds; fingertips cigarette-stained; no hepatosplenomegaly; no increase in JVP; no leg edema.

Labs CBC: elevated hematocrit. Elevated glucose (154 mg/dL); hypercholesterolemia; hypertriglyceridemia; BUN and creatinine normal; LFTs normal. ECG: no signs of ischemia or infarction.

Imaging CXR: calcification of aortic knob, left ventricular hypertrophy. Echo: no segmental wall abnormalities.

Gross Pathology Atherosclerotic narrowing of coronary arteries.

Treatment Adjust timing of nitrate administration in order to have an 8-hour period free of nitroglycerin. Consider alternating with beta-blockers, calcium-channel-blocking agents, or other coronary vasodilators.

Discussion Tolerance is manifested as a poor response to a previously effective dose of nitroglycerin. **Increasing the dosage does not yield relief** of symptoms. The use of other agents, shorter-acting nitroglycerin formulations, or intervals free of nitroglycerin dosing can be tried in an attempt to regain sensitivity to the nitrate. Tolerance and headaches are the main drawbacks of nitrate use for the treatment of angina. Progression of coronary artery disease must always be considered with increasing nitroglycerin requirements.

ID/CC A 56-year-old male comes to the cardiology unit for evaluation of **ringing in his ears** (TINNITUS), **dizziness, GI distress** (nausea, vomiting, and diarrhea), and **headaches**.

HPI He also complains of **blurred vision** and **impaired hearing**. The patient had an MI 1 year ago and has been receiving oral **quinidine** antiarrhythmic therapy.

PE VS: **bradycardia** (HR 55); BP normal (BP 110/70). PE: fundus-copic exam normal but **accommodation impaired; skin flushed**; hands show fine **tremors**; no heart murmurs; lungs clear; abdomen soft and nontender with no masses; no peritoneal signs.

Labs CBC: normal. Lytes: normal. ECG: **widened QRS complex and prolonged Q-T interval**.

Imaging CXR: no pulmonary edema.

Treatment Monitor ECG and vital signs; change to different antiarrhythmic drug. Treat cardiotoxic effects with sodium lactate.

Discussion Quinidine, procainamide, and disopyramide are class IA antiar-rhythmics that act by **blocking sodium channels, increasing the effective refractory period**. They are used for both atrial and ventricular arrhythmias. All these agents have low therapeutic-toxic ratios and may produce severe adverse reactions. **Cinchonism** is commonly produced by drugs that are cinchona derivatives, such as quinidine and quinine. The effects may occur with only one dose.

ID/CC A 73-year-old white widow visits her cardiologist complaining of **difficulty moving her bowels** for the past week; she also reports **facial flushing**.

HPI She had been regular until she began taking **verapamil** for an irregular heart beat 1 month ago.

PE VS: heart rate normal; BP normal; no fever. PE: in no acute distress; no pallor; left eye cataract; no neck masses; no lymphadenopathy; lungs clear; cardiac exam normal; abdomen soft and nondistended; no palpable masses; no peritoneal signs; mild lower leg **edema**.

Labs CBC/Lytes/UA: normal. BUN, glucose, LFTs normal; no hypercalcemia (may produce constipation); normal levels of 5-hydroxyindoleacetic acid (vs. carcinoid syndrome, which may also produce facial flushing but not constipation).

Imaging CXR: within normal limits for age. KUB: moderate amount of stool; no sign of obstruction.

Treatment Increase fluids in diet, regular exercise, fruits, high-bulk foods, or bulk laxatives. If persistent, change to another calcium channel blocker.

Discussion Verapamil is one of the agents that block voltage-dependent calcium channels, consequently reducing muscle contractility. Verapamil acts more specifically on myocardial fibers than on arteriolar smooth muscle. It is widely used as an antihypertensive, as an antiarrhythmic agent, and for treatment of angina pectoris. **Constipation** is a common side effect; other side effects include dizziness, facial **flushing**, hyperprolactinemia, and peripheral edema.

ID/CC A 19-year-old female is admitted to the internal medicine ward because of **generalized desquamation** of the skin, high **fever**, and painful **ulcers and bullae in her eyes and vagina**.

HPI She adds that **swallowing** is extremely **painful**. For the past week, she has been on oral **sulfonamides** for a urinary tract infection.

PE VS: **fever** (39.2°C). PE: painful **mucosal ulcerations** in conjunctiva, nose, mouth, oropharynx, and vagina; eyelids swollen and erythematous; **generalized, symmetric rash** on skin with **macules, papules, vesicles**, and **bullae** (multiple primary skin lesions) as well as areas of denudation (epidermis completely separated from dermis) on palms, soles, and extremities.

Gross Pathology Biopsy distinguishes from toxic epidermal necrolysis, pemphigus, and pemphigoid.

Micro Pathology Dermal edema with perivascular inflammatory infiltrate and epidermal separation in bullae showing necrotic and hemorrhagic areas.

Treatment Hospitalization, discontinue sulfa drug, prophylactic antibiotics (due to increased risk of infections acquired through large areas of denuded skin), barrier nursing, antihistamines. Steroids have not been demonstrated to be effective.

Discussion Also called **erythema multiforme major**, Stevens–Johnson syndrome is a grave, acute, and sometimes fatal disease with generalized skin **desquamation** and severe **ulcers and bullae** on at least two mucosal surfaces, including the genitalia, mouth, conjunctiva, nose, or lips. The use of sulfa drugs (bacteriostatic antibiotics, which are PABA antimetabolites that inhibit dihydropteroate synthase) is a common precipitating factor. Other drugs implicated are **phenytoin**, penicillins and barbiturates.

ID/CC A 26-year-old obsessive-compulsive female comes to the family medicine clinic to have her 5-year-old daughter checked by a dermatologist because of **itching and scaling of her skin**.

HPI The mother is very thin and fears that her daughter will not gain enough weight, so she has given her **cod-liver oil** (rich in vitamin A) **four times a day for the past nine months**. The child complains of **fatigue, headaches**, and **bone pain**.

PE Funduscopic exam reveals **papilledema** (pseudotumor cerebri); localized areas of hair loss (ALOPECIA); very **dry skin** with **scaling** areas on back and extremities; **hyperkeratosis** on medial side of soles of feet; **liver** moderately **enlarged** but not painful.

Labs Increased levels of vitamin A in serum.

Imaging XR, long bones and spine: **cortical hyperostosis; demineralization; premature closure of epiphyses**.

Treatment Discontinue administration of vitamin A-containing supplement.

Discussion Together with vitamins D, E, and K, vitamin A is one of the fat-soluble vitamins, which means that the body stores them and does not eliminate them as quickly as it does water-soluble vitamins. Vitamin A (RETINOL) is derived from carotenes and is a constituent of retinal pigments (RHODOPSIN). Vitamin A is necessary for the integrity of all epithelial cells. **Deficiency of vitamin A produces night blindness** and **xerophthalmia**. Vitamin A is mainly found in meat, liver, fish, and dairy products.

ID/CC A 32-year-old male who works as a professional weight lifter comes to the family medicine clinic for evaluation of **impotence** for the past 4 months.

HPI His girlfriend reports increasingly **aggressive** and **labile behavior**. He has a history of multiple cycles of oral and injectable **anabolic steroid abuse**.

PE VS: **borderline hypertension**. PE: young, muscular male; androgenic **alopecia; acne; gynecomastia; testicular atrophy**.

Labs CBC/Lytes: normal. AST and ALT normal; **hyperglycemia** (145 mg/dL); BUN and creatinine normal; decreased HDL; increased LDL; **oligospermia** on semen analysis.

Imaging CXR: normal. XR, long bones and spine: normal calcification.

Treatment Discontinue androgens.

Discussion Anabolic steroids are widely abused by weight lifters, other athletes, and the lay public. Although androgens increase muscle mass significantly, they produce only slight increases in strength. Numerous side effects have been reported, including **hepatic neoplasia, glucose intolerance, decreased HDL-C levels, hypertension, testicular atrophy and oligospermia, virilization and amenorrhea, acne**, and **alopecia**. Other consequences of androgen abuse include mood disturbances and **irritability** that may result in **aggressive behavior** and injury to others.

ID/CC A 46-year-old female comes to the medical clinic for an evaluation of **weight gain, roundness of her face**, and epigastric pain that is relieved by eating (peptic ulcer).

HPI She had been suffering from chronic, itchy blisters in the mouth that came and went, leaving painful ulcers together with large bullae on all four extremities and on her chest and lower back (PEMPHIGUS), for which she has been taking **high-dose prednisone** for several months.

PE VS: **hypertension** (BP 145/95); no fever. PE: **moon facies, acne, buffalo hump, truncal obesity, striae, increased facial hair** (HIRSUTISM), and **ecchymoses** on distal extremities.

Labs CBC: leukocytosis with **lymphopenia. Hyperglycemia.** Lytes: **hypokalemia.** UA: glycosuria.

Imaging XR, spine and long bones: generalized **osteoporosis.**

Treatment Switch to methotrexate, azathioprine, dapsone, or nicotinamide. Corticosteroids should be tapered down.

Discussion Of the causes of Cushing's syndrome, iatrogenesis is the most common. Steroids produce a lysosomal membrane stabilization, blocking leukotriene formation from arachidonic acid, blocking the action of phospholipase A, and inhibiting cyclooxygenase activity (decreased prostaglandin formation). Because of this, steroids are used in a number of settings, such as acute inflammation, anaphylaxis, allergy states, and immune suppression as well as for the treatment of Addison's disease.

CUSHING'S SYNDROME—IATROGENIC

ID/CC	A 32-year-old woman comes for her first gynecologic visit.
HPI	On routine pelvic exam a vaginal **mass** is felt. The **patient's mother took an estrogen compound** (DES) during pregnancy as treatment for threatened abortion.
PE	Well developed with breast tissue appropriate to age; pubic and axillary hair normal; on bimanual pelvic examination a **hard, ulcerated mass** is felt on posterior **wall of upper vagina**; iodine staining of vaginal wall shows patches of decreased uptake by cells (due to adenosis).
Labs	CBC/Lytes/UA: normal. Hormonal screen and LFTs do not disclose any abnormality.
Imaging	Hysterosalpingogram: injection of contrast into uterine cavity reveals T-shaped uterus and cervical incompetence.
Micro Pathology	Biopsy by colposcopy shows glandular epithelium in upper part of vagina with squamous metaplasia (ADENOSIS). Biopsy of the ulcerated mass shows **clear-cell adenocarcinoma of vagina**.
Treatment	Surgery; radiation.
Discussion	Diethylstilbestrol is a synthetic estrogen that was used some 30 to 35 years ago for the prevention of a threatened abortion. The daughters of patients thus treated before the 18th week of pregnancy may present with an alteration in the development of the embryonic transition between the urogenital canal and paramesonephric system, producing persistence of the müllerian glands on the upper vagina and giving rise to adenosis and clear cell adenocarcinoma that is usually asymptomatic and discovered incidentally. Other side effects include transverse vaginal septum, developmental uterine abnormalities, and cervical incompetence. In males DES may be associated with genital tract abnormalities.

ID/CC	A 17-year-old white female student who is learning how to inject herself with **insulin** is found **unconscious** by her desk.
HPI	The patient suffered from weight loss, polyuria, polydipsia, and polyphagia for several months and was recently diagnosed with **juvenile-onset diabetes mellitus**. She has been meticulous in self-administering insulin injections but often injects larger doses of insulin than prescribed (overdosing is common at the beginning of treatment).
PE	VS: **tachycardia** (HR 96); **hypotension** (BP 100/50); no fever. PE: **skin cold and moist**; patient **stuporous** with hyporeflexia; negative Babinski's sign; responsive only to painful stimuli; cardiopulmonary exam normal; no hepatomegaly; no splenomegaly; no peritoneal signs.
Labs	**Severe hypoglycemia.** Lytes: potassium and magnesium levels sharply decreased (HYPOKALEMIA, HYPOMAGNESEMIA). BUN and creatinine normal; increased serum levels of insulin with normal C-peptide levels.
Imaging	CT, head: no intracranial pathology demonstrated to account for the stuporous state.
Treatment	Administer IV 50% glucose or IM glucagon after drawing baseline blood sample. Follow serum glucose levels for several hours; monitor and treat electrolyte imbalances.
Discussion	With the administration of insulin, blood glucose levels are lowered by direct stimulation of cellular uptake. Glucose uptake is accompanied by a shift of magnesium and potassium into the cell. A severe hypoglycemic coma may result from an insulin overdose, which can produce **permanent neurologic damage or death**.

ID/CC A 36-year-old female oboe player is brought by ambulance to the emergency room because of gradual numbness and **weakness on the left side of her face and arm** along with **headache** and dizziness.

HPI She is **obese** and **smokes** one pack of cigarettes a day. She is currently taking **oral contraceptive pills** (OCPs).

PE VS: normal. PE: patient conscious, oriented, and able to speak; **gaze is deviated to the right**; funduscopic exam does not show papilledema, hypertension, or diabetic retinopathy; lungs clear; abdomen soft and nontender; no peritoneal signs; **left arm and leg weakness with hyporeflexia**.

Labs CBC/Lytes: normal. **Hyperlipidemia**; BUN and creatinine normal; RPR negative; protein C and protein S negative. ECG: normal.

Imaging CT, head: negative. Arteriography: thrombotic cerebral arterial occlusion.

Treatment Intensive care treatment and surveillance for stroke in evolution. Evaluate anticoagulation, discontinue OCPs.

Discussion Oral contraceptive pills are a very popular method of birth control. There are many OCP preparations; most consist of a combination of estrogens and progestins which, when taken daily, selectively inhibit pituitary function to prevent ovulation. The most severe complication is an **increased incidence of vascular thrombotic events**, either cerebral or myocardial. Other side effects include nausea, acne, weight gain, psychological depression, cholestatic jaundice, increased incidence of vaginal infections, headaches, and breakthrough bleeding. OCPs should be used cautiously in patients with asthma, diabetes, liver disease, and hypertension.

ID/CC	A **55-year-old, postmenopausal** white **female** complains of **nausea, headaches, weight gain, and breast tenderness**.
HPI	She was placed on **estrogen** 6 months ago and is also taking **calcium** and **vitamin D**. There is no history of breast, uterine, or ovarian cancer in her family.
PE	VS: normal. PE: mild tenderness to palpation over lumbar vertebrae; breast exam reveals diffuse tenderness without any palpable masses; no axillary lymphadenopathy.
Labs	Lipid profile reveals decreased LDL, increased HDL, and elevated triglycerides.
Imaging	DEXA: **osteopenia** in thoracolumbar vertebral bodies.
Treatment	**Symptomatic control of minor side effects** (as in this patient); if estrogen supplementation is contraindicated or complicated by severe refractory side effects, consider alternative medications for osteoporosis prophylaxis (e.g., calcitonin).
Discussion	Hormone replacement therapy is an effective prophylaxis against primary and secondary osteoporosis (due to hypogonadism, glucocorticoid excess, immobilization, hyperthyroidism, diabetes mellitus, or primary hyperparathyroidism). **Estrogen supplementation** is the first choice for prevention and treatment of osteoporosis in women who are postmenopausal. The mechanism of action is thought to be **decreasing bone resorption** by inhibiting the synthesis of interleukins such as IL-6 as well as retarding the bone-resorbing effects of PTH. Estrogen is contraindicated in **pregnancy, breast cancer**, or **active hepatitis**. Side effects include **breast tenderness, migraines**, and **vaginal bleeding/spotting**. Long-term adverse effects include **gallstones, breast cancer**, and **thrombophlebitis**. Estrogen alone also increases the risk of **endometrial cancer**, and progesterone is often added to decrease this risk.

ID/CC	A **53-year-old, postmenopausal white female** presents to the out-patient clinic with questions regarding "that bone disease" and requests a bone density scan.
HPI	She drinks at least three cups of **coffee and smokes** a pack of cigarettes daily. She is married with two children. There is no history of alcohol abuse, corticosteroid use, or osteoporosis among immediate family members. She **strongly refuses any oral prophylactic hormone therapy**.
PE	VS: normal. PE: unremarkable.
Imaging	DEXA: mild **osteopenia**.
Treatment	**Calcium** and **vitamin D supplementation**; regular **exercise and a balanced diet**; counsel on **fall prevention** and **smoking cessation**; also discuss alternative therapy with **calcitonin**, and **selective estrogen receptor modulators**.
Discussion	Osteoporosis is a bone disease characterized by a decrease in bone density. It is classically a disease of **elderly, thin, postmenopausal Caucasian** or **Asian females** and commonly causes hip and vertebral fractures. Hip fractures can occur secondary to a **fall** but also result from repetitive stress on the hip during intensive exercise programs. **Smoking** increases the risk of osteoporosis, but **caffeine** intake is now believed to have minor or no effect on bone density or fractures. Low to moderate intake of **alcohol** is beneficial, as it increases estrogen levels. **Multiparity** is protective. Calcium is believed to **decrease bone resorption**, probably by inhibiting PTH secretion, but is far less potent than **estrogen** in preventing osteoporosis. Metabolites of **vitamin D** increase the intestinal absorption of calcium, and the most active metabolite, **calcitriol**, or (1,25) OH_2 vitamin D, stimulates bone formation via osteoblasts.

ID/CC	A **67-year-old, postmenopausal white female** presents with **weakness, muscular twitching**, and a nagging **retrosternal heartburn**.
HPI	She was placed on **estrogen** and **alendronate therapy** 6 months ago following the diagnosis of a **spinal compression fracture** secondary to advanced osteoporosis. She is **not on** any **calcium or vitamin D supplementation**.
PE	VS: normal. PE: carpopedal spasm noted on inflating BP cuff (TROUSSEAU'S SIGN); facial twitching noted on tapping anterior to the tragus (CHOVSTEK'S SIGN); spinal kyphosis and protuberant abdomen.
Labs	Lytes: **hypocalcemia. Elevated PTH levels.**
Treatment	**Calcium replacement**; advise to **take alendronate in upright posture** to reduce reflux and risk of esophagitis; H_2 blockers or proton pump inhibitors for concomitant or exacerbated peptic ulcer disease/GERD.
Discussion	Bisphosphonates such as **alendronate** and **pamidronate** increase bone mass by decreasing bone resorption. Side effects include **hypocalcemia, increased PTH levels**, and **upper GI irritation/esophageal ulceration** when given orally. Other medications given for osteoporosis include **raloxifene**, a **selective estrogen receptor modulator (SERM)**, and **calcitonin**. Calcitonin causes increases in bone density (not as much as seen with bisphosphonates) and is a safe alternative to estrogen. Side effects include nasal irritation when administered as a nasal spray.

ENDOCRINOLOGY

ID/CC A **50-year-old white male** presents with **decreased libido, progressive impotence, fatigue**, and **muscle weakness**.

HPI He underwent a **transsphenoidal hypophysectomy** for a **large pituitary tumor** 2 months ago. He is currently on hormone replacement therapy with thyroxine and corticosteroids.

PE VS: normal. PE: bilateral **breast enlargement** (GYNECOMASTIA), **bilateral testicular atrophy**, and **loss of facial and pubic hair**.

Labs **Decreased serum testosterone level; decreased serum LH and FSH.**

Treatment **Testosterone replacement** via either a transdermal testosterone patch or a pill; long-term use of testosterone produces subjective improvement in mood, energy, libido, muscle mass, and sexual function.

Discussion **Hypogonadism** or **testosterone deficiency** is either congenital or acquired. Causes are categorized as either **primary** (hypergonadotropic, high FSH/LH levels) or **secondary** (hypogonadotropic, low FSH/LH levels). The most common congenital cause of primary hypogonadism is Klinefelter's syndrome. Acquired causes include trauma, surgery, testicular torsion, irradiation, chemotherapy, alcoholism, and aging. Secondary hypogonadism is associated with disorders such as Kallmann's and Prader–Willi Syndromes or with pituitary tumors or trauma. Side effects of testosterone include **itching** and **local irritation** (when given topically) and **liver dysfunction** and a **decrease in HDL** (when given orally). Testosterone is contraindicated in men with prostatic carcinoma.

ID/CC A **37-year-old obese male** presents with recent worsening of his anginal symptoms.

HPI He suffers from **coronary artery disease** and regularly takes anti-anginal medications. One month ago, he began to take **Metabolife 356** for weight loss and to "increase his energy level." He drinks **three cups of coffee a day**.

PE VS: borderline **hypertension** (BP 150/100). PE: unremarkable.

Labs ECG: normal.

Imaging CXR: normal.

Treatment **Stop ephedrine** containing supplement and educate on risks of unsupervised use of herbal/alternative medicines; evaluate for worsening coronary artery disease if symptoms do not abate after stopping the supplement.

Discussion **Herbal supplements** as alternative medicines are currently in widespread use. Over 20% of the general population use herbal supplements for health, but fewer than 50% of those taking supplements tell their physician. **Metabolife 356** is a combination of many active herbs that is sold over the counter as a weight-loss supplement. One of the ingredients in Metabolife 356 is **ephedrine (Ma Huang)**, a sympathomimetic drug that stimulates the sympathetic nervous system and is synergistic with **caffeine**. The adverse effects of ephedrine include **increased blood pressure, palpitations, chest pain, psychosis, tremor, insomnia, dry mouth**, and **cardiomyopathy** linked to chronic use.

ID/CC	A **36-year-old white morbidly obese woman** presents to her primary care physician, seeking help with losing weight.
HPI	She has tried various diets and exercise programs with no success.
PE	VS: normal. PE: morbidly obese.
Labs	CBC/Lytes: normal. Lipid panel, LFTs, TSH normal.
Treatment	**Orlistat** or **sibutramine** in combination with a structured diet and exercise program.
Discussion	Obesity contributes to **atherosclerosis, CAD, hyperlipidemia, hypertension, and type II diabetes**. Anti-obesity drugs currently on the market include **orlistat** and **sibutramine**. They are indicated for weight loss and maintenance in conjunction with a calorie-reduced diet in patients with a body mass index ≥ 30. Orlistat is a **lipase inhibitor** that acts in the GI tract and **blocks the absorption of dietary fat**. The most common adverse effects are GI-related and include spotting, flatus, and fatty stools. Absorption of lipid-soluble vitamins (e.g., vitamin K) or medications (e.g., griseofulvin) may be decreased. Sibutramine treats obesity through **appetite suppression**; it acts centrally by blocking serotonin and norepinephrine reuptake. Adverse effects include headache, dry mouth, constipation, insomnia, and a **substantial increase in blood pressure and heart rate in some patients**. Unlike the discontinued drug fenfluramine, sibutramine does not cause pulmonary hypertension or cardiac valve dysfunction. Sibutramine is contraindicated in patients on MAO inhibitors or SSRIs (may precipitate **serotonin syndrome**), in those with CHF/CAD, and in those with hepatic dysfunction (the drug is metabolized by **cytochrome P450**).

ID/CC A 64-year-old male with **metastatic lung cancer** is seen with complaints of **severe bone pain, anorexia**, and **cachexia**.

HPI He spends most of his time in bed because of profound weakness and chronic nausea.

PE VS: **mild fever** (38.0°C); **tachycardia** (HR 110); **underweight** (45 kg, body mass index 17). PE: **cachectic; sunken eyes; prominent skin wrinkles/folds; visible loss of significant skeletal muscle mass**.

Labs CBC: lymphopenia. Lytes: **hypokalemia; hypochloremia**. ABGs: **metabolic alkalosis. Decreased albumin and prealbumin/ transthyretin.**

Treatment Treat with **megestrol acetate or dronabinol** to increase appetite; adequate palliative pain medications.

Discussion **Cachexia/anorexia syndrome** is characterized by progressive weight loss, lipolysis, loss of muscle mass, anorexia, diarrhea, and fever in patients with end-stage cancer or AIDS. Some drugs that have proven effective in improving appetite and treating cachexia include **megestrol acetate** and **dronabinol**. Megestrol is a synthetic progesterone that stimulates the appetite, resulting in weight gain and recovery of muscle mass. It is relatively nontoxic. Side effects are rare and include **altered menses with unpredictable bleeding** and **mild edema**. Dronabinol, a synthetic **tetrahydrocannabinol (THC)**, is the active component in **marijuana** and is used to treat nausea and vomiting associated with cancer chemotherapy as well as to stimulate appetite. Side effects are due mainly to the psychoactive effects of the drug and include dizziness, ataxia, hallucinations/psychosis, tachycardia, hypertension, and URI symptoms.

ID/CC A 39-year-old male presents to his family doctor because of increasing embarrassment and concern over **breast enlargement**.

HPI The patient has a long history of burning epigastric pain on awakening in the mornings and between meals that decreases with food and antacids (peptic ulcer disease), for which he has been taking **cimetidine**. Directed questioning reveals that he has also been suffering from **hallucinations** and **impotence**.

PE VS: normal. PE: cardiovascular, neurologic, and abdominal examination fail to reveal any pathology; moderate bilateral growth of breast tissue; **testes** somewhat **hypotrophic**; rectal exam negative for prostatic enlargement.

Labs CBC/Lytes/UA: normal.

Imaging CXR/KUB: normal.

Treatment Switch to other histamine receptor antagonists, such as raniti-dine or famotidine.

Discussion All the H_2 blockers are well tolerated, although cimetidine is associated with several side effects, particularly **reversible gynecomastia**. H_2 blockers produce an **increase in serum pro-lactin levels** (especially ranitidine) and alter estrogen metabo-lism in men (have anti-androgenic properties). Other side effects include headache, confusion, low sperm counts, and hematologic abnormalities (thrombocytopenia may enhance hy-poprothrombinemic effect of oral anticoagulants). They have been largely supplanted by newer H_2 receptor blockers without many of these side effects.

ID/CC	A 58-year-old female comes to the emergency room because of acute, burning **epigastric pain** accompanied by nausea and **vomiting** of **bright red blood**.
HPI	She is a chronic sufferer of rheumatoid arthritis and has taken 650 mg of **aspirin** every 8 hours for the past 4 years to control her pain.
PE	VS: **tachycardia** (HR 98); hypotension (BP 110/60); no fever. PE: **pallor**; anxiety; abdomen shows **tenderness on deep palpation in epigastrium**; no rigidity, guarding, or rebound tenderness; no masses palpable; no focal neurologic signs; hands show characteristic rheumatoid characteristics.
Labs	CBC: low hemoglobin and hematocrit. ABGs/Lytes: mild metabolic alkalosis with hypokalemia (due to vomiting of hydrochloric acid).
Imaging	Endoscopy: gastric mucosa markedly hyperemic with hemorrhagic spotting and zones of recent hemorrhage; no ulcer or tumor observed.
Treatment	Discontinue offending agent (salicylates); start mucosal protectors, antacids, proton pump inhibitors, or H_2 receptor blockers.
Discussion	Hemorrhagic gastritis is seen in individuals who take drugs that may cause damage to gastric mucosa, such as aspirin, NSAIDs, steroids, and alcohol. Critically ill patients, such as those with burns, sepsis, cranial trauma, and coagulation defects, may also bleed from the stomach. Acetylsalicylic acid (aspirin) acetylates and irreversibly inhibits cyclooxygenase I and II to prevent conversion of arachidonic acid to prostaglandins.

HEMORRHAGIC GASTRITIS—DRUG-INDUCED

ID/CC A 64-year-old female is brought to the emergency room because of the development of high fever, **marked jaundice**, weakness, profound fatigue, and **darkening of her urine**.

HPI She has undergone many surgical procedures **under general anesthesia** (halothane) over the past 2 years, including a colpoperineoplasty, an endometrial biopsy, a femoral hernia repair, and, 4 weeks ago, a total hip replacement. After each surgery, the patient developed a low-grade fever within a few days.

PE VS: **tachycardia** (HR 93); hypotension (BP 100/55); fever (39.2°C). PE: **marked weakness**; diaphoresis; patient appears **toxic**; profound **jaundice**; liver edge palpable 3 cm below costal margin and tender.

Labs CBC: marked **leukocytosis** (18,500) with **eosinophilia** (18%) (allergic reaction). Hypoglycemia; **AST and ALT markedly elevated; elevated alkaline phosphatase and bilirubin**.

Gross Pathology Massive centrolobular hepatic necrosis with fatty change.

Treatment Monitor liver function; assess bilirubin, glucose levels, and PT. Provide intensive supportive care for possible hepatic failure and encephalopathy. Treat hypoglycemia with glucose, treat bleeding with fresh frozen plasma, and use lactulose to prevent encephalopathy.

Discussion All inhaled anesthetics cause a decrease in hepatic blood flow, but rarely does this result in permanent derangement of liver function tests. Nonetheless, hydrocarbon drugs that include halothane are considered hepatotoxic. Most commonly, such drugs produce elevated LFTs, but they may also cause postoperative jaundice and hepatitis. Rarely does fulminant hepatic failure result, but such failure carries a 50% mortality rate. Occurrence is normally 4 to 6 weeks after halothane exposure. Middle-aged, obese women with several halothane exposures within closely spaced intervals are most at risk.

ID/CC A 52-year-old HIV-positive male who was diagnosed with **tuberculosis** and started on **isoniazid** (INH) therapy 8 months ago presents with **jaundice**.

HPI The patient's isoniazid therapy was uneventful until 2 weeks ago, when he began to appear jaundiced. He also complains of **lack of strength and sensation in his feet**.

PE VS: normal. PE: patient appears lethargic; yellowed sclera and discoloration of skin; funduscopic exam normal; moderate, nontender hepatomegaly; decreased strength and diminished perception of light touch in feet.

Labs Moderately **increased AST, ALT**, and **bilirubin**.

Imaging US: generalized mild enlargement of liver with no focal lesions.

Treatment More than a two- to threefold increase in AST and ALT warrants cessation of INH use. Also stop rifampin if it is part of multidrug therapy for tuberculosis. Substitution with second-line antitubercular agents (e.g., fluoroquinolones, aminoglycosides) may be required. Mild derangement of liver function warrants close monitoring while treatment with INH is continued. Coadministration of pyridoxine with INH is recommended to prevent and possibly ameliorate peripheral neurotoxicity.

Discussion Isoniazid (isonicotinic acid hydrazide) decreases the synthesis of mycolic acids and is the bactericidal drug of choice for tuberculosis prophylaxis. It is used as combination therapy for eradication of *Mycobacterium tuberculosis*. Chronic use is associated with **hepatitis, peripheral neuritis**, disulfiram-like reaction, and **systemic lupus erythematosus**. INH competes with pyridoxine for the enzyme apotryptophanase, thus producing a deficiency of pyridoxine. The administration of pyridoxine can prevent some central and peripheral nervous system effects. The risk for hepatitis and multilobular necrosis is greater in alcoholics and older persons.

ID/CC	A 22-year-old female presents to the ER with severe abdominal colic and a history of **profuse watery diarrhea** of several days' duration.
HPI	She also complains of **dizziness** and a **desire to lose weight** (directed questioning discloses that she has been taking **magnesium sulfate** intermittently).
PE	VS: **hypotension** (BP 80/45); no fever. PE: **skin shriveled; bowel sounds hyperactive**; oliguric and lethargic.
Labs	Lytes: hypokalemia; hyponatremia; hyperchloremia. ABGs: normal anion gap metabolic acidosis.
Treatment	Discontinue laxatives and offer counseling. Give IV glucose and electrolytes to restore fluid balance.
Discussion	Laxative abuse remains a common way people attempt to lose weight; abuse is also common among psychiatric patients. Laxatives can interfere with the absorption of several medications, such as tetracycline and calcium supplements. Laxatives may act by irritating the mucosa, through direct neuronal stimulation, via an osmotic increase in the water content of stool, through softening of stool by a detergent-like action, or by forming bulk. Continued abuse may lead to melanosis coli, colonic neuronal degeneration, and the "lazy intestine syndrome." Patients with chronic constipation abuse laxatives to the point of being dependent on them for evacuation.

ID/CC	A 28-year-old white female has surgery due to perforated appendicitis with peritonitis; 10 days postoperatively she develops fever, abdominal cramping, and **diarrhea with pus and mucus**.
HPI	Her postoperative recovery was unremarkable until the onset of diarrhea. She had **received continuous parenteral antibiotics (clindamycin)**.
PE	VS: fever; tachycardia; tachypnea. PE: moderate dehydration; mild abdominal tenderness with no signs of peritoneal irritation; surgical wound normal.
Labs	CBC: leukocytosis. Stool culture reveals gram-positive rods, *Clostridium difficile*; **presence of toxin in stool**.
Imaging	Sigmoidoscopy: mucosal hyperemia, ulcers, and **pseudomembranes**.
Gross Pathology	Mucosa hyperemic and swollen; epithelial ulcerations covered by yellowish plaques (pseudomembranes) and fibrinous exudate.
Micro Pathology	Fibrinous exudate with pseudomembrane formation; ulceration of superficial epithelium; neutrophilic infiltrate with necrotic debris.
Treatment	Cessation of offending antibiotic; give **metronidazole** or oral vancomycin.
Discussion	Pseudomembranous colitis is defined as acute inflammation of the colon in patients taking antibiotics, specifically **clindamycin** or ampicillin, due to **overgrowth of *C. difficile***; it is characterized by formation of **pseudomembranes**. Clindamycin acts by blocking protein synthesis at the 50S ribosomal unit. Its main clinical indication is for life-threatening infections with **anaerobes**.
Atlas Link	UCVI PG-PH-031

PSEUDOMEMBRANOUS COLITIS

ID/CC A 6-year-old boy is brought by his parents to the emergency room in a **comatose state**.

HPI The child had been suffering from **chickenpox** and had been given **aspirin** by the family physician for fever.

PE VS: **fever**. PE: comatose child with **papulovesicular rash** all over body; fundus shows **marked papilledema**; no icterus; moderate hepatomegaly; asterixis.

Labs **Marked hypoglycemia; increased blood ammonia concentration; elevated AST and ALT; prolonged PT**; serum bilirubin normal. LP (done after lowering raised intracranial pressure): normal CSF.

Imaging CT: findings suggestive of **generalized cerebral edema**.

Gross Pathology Severe cerebral edema; acute hepatic necrosis.

Micro Pathology Liver biopsy reveals microvesicular steatosis with little or no inflammation; electron microscopy shows marked mitochondrial abnormalities.

Treatment Specific therapy not available. Supportive measures include lactulose to control hyperammonemia, fresh frozen plasma to replenish clotting factors, mannitol or dexamethasone to lower increased intracranial pressure, and mechanical ventilation. Exchange transfusion; dialysis.

Discussion Although the cause of the highly lethal Reye's syndrome (hepatoencephalopathy) is unknown, epidemiologic evidence strongly links this disorder with outbreaks of viral disease, especially influenza B and chickenpox. Epidemiologic evidence has also prompted the Surgeon General and the American Academy of Pediatrics Committee on Infectious Diseases to recommend that **salicylates not be given to children with chickenpox or influenza B**.

ID/CC	A 51-year-old chemical engineer who manages the production line at a large **petrochemical plant** comes to his family doctor for a yearly checkup; he is asymptomatic but is found to have **microscopic** painless **hematuria**.
HPI	He is a **heavy smoker** and has been working at the production plant over a period of 25 years.
PE	VS: normal. PE: strongly built male with gray hair and smoke discoloration of his mustache and fingertips; a few wheezes heard on lung fields; heart sounds normal; abdominal exam normal; no lymphadenopathy; genitalia normal; rectal exam normal.
Labs	CBC/Lytes: normal. Clinical chemistry and LFTs normal; BUN and creatinine normal. UA: **hematuria**.
Imaging	US: no renoureteral lithiasis; no pelvicalyceal dilatation. Excretory urography: filling defect and rigidity in wall of urinary bladder.
Micro Pathology	Urine cytology shows marked dysplastic and anaplastic transitional cells; cystoscopy and biopsy confirm a **papillary transitional cell carcinoma (TCC) of the bladder**.
Treatment	Surgery, chemotherapy, radiotherapy.
Discussion	The substances 2-amino-1-naphthol and p-diphenylamine are the two carcinogens that are presumed to be involved in the genesis of transitional cell bladder cancer in individuals exposed to anilines, benzidine, and β-naphthylamines. Saccharin has been shown to induce TCC in rats. Cigarette smoking greatly increases the risk. Heavy caffeine consumption remains a controversial risk factor.

ANILINE DYE CARCINOGENICITY

ID/CC	A **73-year-old** farmer complains of **dry cough** of 2 months' duration together with intermittent **fever, vomiting**, and increasing **dyspnea**.
HPI	He had a squamous cell carcinoma lesion surgically removed from his nose several months ago and received chemotherapy with **bleomycin**.
PE	Healed skin flap on left nasal fossa; no local lymphadenopathy; multiple freckles and solar dermatitis on scalp; scattered lung **rales and wheezing; soles of feet** show painful, erythematous areas with **skin thickening**.
Labs	CBC/Lytes: normal. LFTs normal; BUN and creatinine normal. PFTs: decreased FEV_1 and FVC with normal FEV_1/FVC ratio.
Imaging	CXR: bilateral pulmonary infiltrates but no evidence of metastatic disease.
Micro Pathology	Lung biopsy shows interstitial pneumonitis with fibrosis and bronchiolar squamous metaplasia.
Treatment	Steroids, antibiotics, discontinue bleomycin.
Discussion	Bleomycin is an antibiotic produced by *Streptomyces verticillus* that acts by DNA fragmentation. It is used in a variety of epidermoid and testicular cancers. Fever and chills may ensue with the administration of the drug by any of the parenteral routes available (it is not active orally). It has very little marrow toxicity and almost no immune suppression, but the keratinized areas of the body may suffer from hypertrophy and nail pigmentation. **Pulmonary fibrosis** is a side effect that characteristically arises in older patients and in those with preexisting lung disease.

ID/CC	A 20-year-old male with testicular cancer presents to his oncologist with a pronounced **decrease in bilateral auditory acuity**.
HPI	His last two chemotherapy sessions were administered by an intern who only recently arrived at the municipal hospital.
PE	VS: normal. PE: auditory testing shows bilateral **neurosensory deficit in the high-frequency range**; lung fields do not show crackles or wheezing; heart sounds rhythmic with no murmurs; abdomen soft with no masses; neurologic exam reveals loss of **proprioception** in feet and diminished sensation in hands and feet (STOCKING-GLOVE PATTERN).
Labs	CBC: normal. Lytes: **hypomagnesemia; hypocalcemia**; hypernatremia; hypokalemia. **BUN and creatinine increased**.
Imaging	CT, head: no intracranial causes of hearing loss revealed.
Treatment	Discontinue cisplatin; replace electrolytes. Pretreatment with amifostine may reduce toxicity.
Discussion	Cisplatin is an effective chemotherapeutic drug that acts like an alkylating agent, cross-linking DNA via the hydrolysis of chloride groups and reaction with platinum. It is used for bladder and testicular cancers as well as for some ovarian tumors. It can produce severe **renal damage** if administered in the absence of abundant hydration. It also causes **CN VIII damage** with permanent deafness. Another side effect is **peripheral neuropathy**.

CISPLATIN SIDE EFFECTS

ID/CC   A 40-year-old male who has been diagnosed with pemphigus vulgaris complains of **dysuria** and **increased urinary frequency**.

HPI   The patient has no history of fever or gross hematuria. He is receiving monthly dexamethasone-**cyclophosphamide pulse therapy**.

PE   VS: normal. PE: no pallor; lungs clear to auscultation; cardiac exam normal; abdomen soft and nontender; no suprapubic masses; no peritoneal signs; no tenderness in costovertebral angle.

Labs   CBC: normocytic, normochromic **anemia**; mild leukopenia and thrombocytopenia. UA: **microscopic hematuria** but no bacteriuria.

Treatment   Maintain good hydration and HCO_3 loading; ϵ-amino caproic acid and mesna may prevent hemorrhagic cystitis.

Discussion   Cyclophosphamide is an alkylating agent that covalently cross-links DNA at guanine N-7 and requires bioactivation by the liver. It is used for lymphomas and for breast and ovarian carcinomas. Complications of cyclophosphamide use include **hemorrhagic cystitis, bladder fibrosis**, and **bladder carcinoma; sterility; alopecia**; and inappropriate ADH secretion. Cyclophosphamide needs to be converted to an active toxic metabolite, **acrolein**, which is responsible for producing hemorrhagic cystitis.

ID/CC	A 24-year-old delivery man for an international courier service currently being treated for **testicular carcinoma** is brought by ambulance to the ER after **fainting while at work**.
HPI	The patient had noticed a painless lump in his right testicle 3 months earlier; a biopsy found testicular carcinoma, for which he was given **doxorubicin** chemotherapy.
PE	VS: **tachycardia** (HR 110); BP normal (118/85). PE: **elevated JVP**; S3 auscultated; **basal rales** in lung fields; **hepatomegaly**; **pitting edema** in lower legs.
Labs	ECG: ST-T changes, premature ventricular contractions; decreased QRS voltage.
Imaging	CXR: cardiomegaly and pulmonary congestion. Echo: dilated cardiomyopathy with reduced ejection fraction.
Gross Pathology	Increase in weight and size of heart with softened, weak walls and dilated chambers (DILATED CARDIOMYOPATHY).
Treatment	Treatment of heart failure due to **dilated cardiomyopathy**. Discontinue doxorubicin.
Discussion	Doxorubicin, also called adriamycin, is an anthracycline antibiotic that binds to DNA and blocks the synthesis of new RNA and/or DNA, thereby blocking cell replication. It is used in the treatment of carcinomas of the ovary, breast, testicle, lung, and thyroid. It is also used in the treatment of many types of sarcomas and hematologic cancers. Side effects are mainly cardiac but may also include alopecia and marrow toxicity (cardiomyopathy associated with doxorubicin is dose-related and irreversible; the mechanisms may be related to the intracellular production of free radicals in myocardium, which can be prevented by dexrazoxane).

DOXORUBICIN CARDIOTOXICITY

ID/CC A **74-year-old female** who recently had hip replacement surgery has been on **postoperative IV heparin** for 5 days for the prevention of possible pulmonary embolism; shortly thereafter, she starts to have black, tarry stools (MELENA, GI BLEEDING), hematuria, and **bleeding from the gums** when brushing her teeth.

HPI She suffers from long-standing cardiac disease and has a **history of deep venous thrombosis**. However, the dose administered was excessive.

PE VS: no fever; **heart rate slightly elevated above baseline**; BP within normal limits but drops when patient stands up (ORTHOSTATIC HYPOTENSION). PE: **pallor**; no signs of cardiac failure; **incision is oozing blood**; venipuncture sites show large **ecchymoses**.

Labs CBC: normocytic, normochromic **anemia** (7.3 mg/dL). **aPTT and PT markedly elevated; platelet count low**.

Imaging CXR: within normal limits for age. XR, hip: no evidence of hematoma formation.

Treatment Stop heparin; for significant bleeding complications, IV **protamine sulfate** is the specific antidote.

Discussion Heparin complexes with **antithrombin III** to form a potent **inactivator of factor Xa** and **inhibitor of the conversion of prothrombin** to thrombin. This complex also inactivates factors IXa, XIa, and XIIa. Its major adverse effect is bleeding, which occurs with a higher incidence in women over age 60. Other adverse effects include hypersensitivity, hyperlipidemia, hyperkalemia, osteoporosis, and, in up to 30% of patients, thrombocytopenia. The severity of thrombocytopenia appears to be dose related and is due to the direct effect of heparin on platelets or to an immunoglobulin that aggregates platelets.

ID/CC	A 9-year-old male is brought to the emergency room after intentionally ingesting half a bottle of **iron tablets** (coated with plum-flavored sugar) 6 hours ago; he now complains of **abdominal pain and diarrhea**.
HPI	He has been feeling weak and lightheaded, with palpitations and a metallic taste in his mouth. He had two episodes of **bluish-green vomit** followed by a large **hematemesis**.
PE	VS: marked **tachycardia** (HR 120); **hypotension** (BP 90/50); no fever. PE: pulse weak; patient is **pale and dehydrated** with cold and clammy skin; lungs clear; abdomen tender to deep palpation, predominantly in epigastrium, with no peritoneal signs; neurologic exam normal; rectal exam discloses black, tarry stool.
Labs	Markedly elevated serum iron levels (> 500 mg/dL). UA: rose-wine-colored urine. ABGs: metabolic acidosis. BUN and creatinine elevated.
Imaging	XR, abdomen: multiple **radiopaque iron tablets** in GI tract from stomach to jejunum. Endoscopy: **diffuse hemorrhagic gastritis** with extensive necrosis and sloughing of mucosa.
Treatment	Gastric lavage with bicarbonate solution (to form ferrous carbonate, which is not absorbed well) or induction of vomiting. Treat acidosis; treat shock with IV fluids and **chelation** therapy with **deferoxamine**.
Discussion	Mortality due to acute iron overdose may reach 25% or more, mainly in children. There may be marked dehydration and shock.

IRON OVERDOSE

ID/CC A 62-year-old female comes to the general oncology unit of the university hospital for **ulceration of the oral mucosa and diarrhea**.

HPI She is being treated for carcinoma of the breast with aggressive methotrexate therapy. Because of impaired renal function, methotrexate toxicity was enhanced. Leucovorin administration did not diminish the cytotoxic effects on normal cells.

PE VS: hypotension (BP 100/50); tachycardia (HR 105). PE: lethargic and dehydrated; oral mucosa and tongue show erythema and shallow ulcers (BUCCAL STOMATITIS); skin rash on volar aspect of forearms.

Labs CBC: **anemia; thrombocytopenia; leukopenia** (myelosuppression). BUN and creatinine elevated.

Treatment The efficacy of leucovorin therapy depends on early administration when methotrexate toxicity is suspected. Give IV dose equal to or greater than the dose of methotrexate.

Discussion Methotrexate binds **reversibly** with dihydrofolate reductase, preventing the synthesis of purine and pyrimidine nucleotides. The toxic effects on proliferating tissues are particularly deleterious to the bone marrow, skin, and GI mucosa. **Leucovorin** "rescue" attenuates some of these toxic effects because it is a metabolically active form of folic acid. For that reason, it does not require reduction by dihydrofolate reductase. Therefore, leucovorin has the capacity to catalyze the one-carbon transfer reactions necessary for purine and pyrimidine biosynthesis.

METHOTREXATE TOXICITY

ID/CC	A 53-year-old woman presents with **dizziness and spontaneous severe bruising**.
HPI	She reports passage of several dark, tarry stools (MELENA). She underwent a valve replacement several months ago and is currently taking **warfarin** (COUMADIN) for anticoagulation prophylaxis. One week ago, she was given **co-trimoxazole** (a sulfa antibiotic) for a "sinus infection," but she neglected to tell her doctor about the Coumadin.
PE	VS: **orthostatic hypotension** (BP 110/70, HR 95 when supine; BP 90/60, HR 110 when erect). PE: extensive ecchymoses and petechiae noted on skin exam; black, tarry guaiac positive stools on rectal exam.
Labs	CBC: **anemia. PT, INR, PTT markedly elevated**.
Treatment	Supportive (blood transfusion and IV fluids); for significant bleeding complications associated with warfarin use (as in this case), withhold warfarin, administer **fresh frozen plasma** and parenteral **vitamin K**, and monitor serial PT/PTT/INR.
Discussion	**Warfarin** is an **anticoagulant** commonly used in patients with **underlying hypercoagulable states, prosthetic cardiac valves, cardiac arrhythmias, DVTs, and pulmonary embolism**. It acts by interfering with the hepatic synthesis of vitamin K-dependent clotting factors, resulting in depletion of factors VII, IX, X, and II. Warfarin is highly **protein bound**, primarily to albumin, and is metabolized by the hepatic **cytochrome P450 enzyme system. Drug interactions** with warfarin are extensive. They include increased effect due to inhibition of metabolism (e.g., amiodarone, cimetidine, co-trimoxazole), possible increased effect due to displacement from albumin (e.g., chloral hydrate, furosemide), and decreased effect due to induction of metabolism (e.g., barbiturates, rifampin).

ID/CC	A 32-year-old male with a prosthetic heart valve complains to his family doctor of **black, tarry stools**.
HPI	He had been receiving **oral warfarin** (COUMADIN) to prevent thrombus formation. Two years ago, he had an **aortic valve replacement** due to destruction of the valve secondary to bacterial endocarditis.
PE	VS: BP normal; pulse rate normal. PE: subconjunctival hemorrhage; bleeding gums; **bruises and petechiae** on arms and legs (generalized bleeding).
Labs	**Stool guaiac positive. UA: hematuria. Markedly elevated PT** (affects extrinsic coagulation pathway).
Treatment	If significant bleeding and volume depletion have occurred, consider fresh frozen plasma and transfusions. Vitamin K may be required.
Discussion	This patient has generalized bleeding, including GI tract bleeding secondary to warfarin treatment. Warfarin compounds inhibit epoxide reductase and hepatic production of the vitamin K-dependent clotting factors (II, VII, IX, and X), interfering with their γ-carboxylation. Only de novo synthesis is affected; therefore, therapy must continue for 2 to 3 days before effects are noted. Effects of warfarin last between 5 and 7 days. Warfarin crosses the placenta and is thus contraindicated in pregnant women.

ID/CC A 45-year-old male who received a **renal transplant** 4 months ago comes to the oncology unit for a follow-up exam complaining of headache and ringing in his ears. He was found to have **hypertension**.

HPI He is currently taking multiple **immunosuppressive** drugs, including **cyclosporine**.

PE VS: **hypertension** (BP 150/110). PE: no jaundice; no pallor; cardiac exam normal; abdomen soft and nontender; no abdominal masses; no peritoneal signs; fine hand **tremors** at rest.

Labs Elevated cyclosporine levels; **elevated BUN and serum creatinine**. Lytes: **hyperkalemia**. UA: **proteinuria**. ECG: peaked T waves (hyperkalemia).

Micro Pathology Renal biopsy reveals presence of tubular lesions (vacuolization), atrophy, edema, microcalcifications, and absence of an acute cellular infiltrate that is characteristic of acute rejection.

Treatment Reduction in cyclosporine dose with serial monitoring.

Discussion Subacute cyclosporine nephrotoxicity is frequently seen in the first few weeks or months after renal transplantation, and it is often unclear whether the renal allograft dysfunction results from acute cellular rejection or cyclosporine toxicity. Renal biopsy is often necessary to guide therapy. Other clinical signs of cyclosporine toxicity include **hyperkalemia, hypertension, tremors, seizures, hirsutism, gingival hypertrophy**, and breast fibroadenomas.

CYCLOSPORINE SIDE EFFECTS

ID/CC A 58-year-old female presents with **persistent fever, chills, headache, weakness**, and **diffuse muscle and bone aches**.

HPI She was diagnosed with **chronic myelocytic leukemia** (CML) a few months ago and is now being treated with oral hydroxyurea and subcutaneous **interferon**.

PE VS: **fever** (39.0°C); **tachycardia** (HR 105). PE: appears fatigued; splenomegaly on abdominal exam.

Labs CBC: **anemia**; mild **leukopenia**; mild **thrombocytopenia**. No blast cells seen.

Treatment Continue interferon therapy as long as side effects are tolerable; monitor for severe **pancytopenia**.

Discussion Interferons are **cytokines** with antiviral, antiproliferative, and immunomodulating properties. They are used to treat chronic hepatitis B, C, or D infection (α2b), condyloma acuminatum (genital warts) due to HPV (α2b, αn3), CML or hairy-cell leukemia (α2a, α2b), Kaposi's sarcoma (α2a, α2b), melanoma (α2b) and chronic granulomatous disease (γ2b). Side effects include **fever, chills, myalgias, fatigue, pancytopenia**, and **neurotoxicity** that presents as **somnolence** and **confusion**. Autoimmune phenomena, including **thyroiditis** (both hypo- and hyperthyroidism), **autoimmune hemolytic anemia**, and **thrombo-cytopenia**, can also occur secondary to interferon use.

ID/CC During ward rounds, a 28-year-old HIV-positive female patient complains that after a period of improvement since her admission 3 days ago, she now feels very sick, with **high fever, marked lightheadedness, headache**, and **myalgias**.

HPI She was admitted because of **cryptococcal meningitis** and was started on **amphotericin B**.

PE VS: tachycardia (HR 93); **hypotension** (BP 90/55); **fever** (39.3°C); **tachypnea**. PE: nuchal rigidity resolved; mental status improved.

Labs CBC: mild **anemia**; normal leukocytes. Lytes: **hypokalemia. BUN and creatinine** moderately **elevated**.

Treatment If the reaction is severe, it may be necessary to lower the dosage of amphotericin B, use a liposomal form, or change to fluconazole. Antipyretics, antihistamines, and corticosteroids may lessen febrile symptoms; heparin can decrease the risk of thrombophlebitis.

Discussion The mechanism of action of amphotericin B is by **binding to ergosterol in fungi** and forming membrane pores. Toxicities include **arrhythmias, chills and fever, hypotension**, and **nephrotoxicity**.

AMPHOTERICIN B TOXICITY

ID/CC   A 31-year-old truck driver visits a health clinic in San Diego complaining of **recurrent infections** (neutropenia), excessive **bleeding** (thrombocytopenia) and malaise, **weakness**, and apathy (anemia).

HPI   He travels south of the border daily and eats and sleeps there. He has had **typhoid fever** three times over the past 5 years, for which he has been treated with high-dose **chloramphenicol**.

PE   VS: no fever; BP normal. PE: marked **pallor**; lungs clear; heart sounds normal; generalized **petechiae**; abdominal and neuro-logic examination unremarkable.

Labs   CBC: **anemia** (Hb 5.7); **leukopenia; thrombocytopenia**.

Imaging   CXR/KUB: within normal limits.

Treatment Blood transfusions, antithymocyte globulin or cyclosporin, marrow transplantation.

Discussion Chloramphenicol is a bacteriostatic antibiotic that acts by inhibiting peptidyl transferase in the 50S ribosomal unit. It is active against anaerobes (abdominal sepsis) and rickettsiae as well as against typhoid fever and meningococcal, streptococcal, and *Haemophilus influenzae* meningitis. **Aplastic anemia** is nonetheless a major problem. Some aplastic cases appear to be related to overdose, while others are related to hypersensitivity to the drug. In infants, it produces the **gray-baby syndrome**. Owing to its potentially fatal side effect of **aplastic anemia**, chloramphenicol is used primarily for serious infections or acute *Salmonella typhi* infection.

ID/CC	A 37-year-old missionary returning home from central **Africa** comes to the tropical medicine department of the local university for an evaluation of **blurred vision** and seeing **"halos" around lights** at night.
HPI	He also complains of marked **itching while showering** and notes that his **hair** has been turning prematurely **gray**. He has been taking weekly doses of **chloroquine** for the suppression of hyperendemic malaria.
PE	"Half-moon-shaped" **corneal deposits** on funduscopic exam; diminished visual acuity bilaterally and **retinal edema** with pigmentation; slight **desquamation of palms of hands**; lungs clear; no heart murmurs; no hepatosplenomegaly; no focal neurologic signs.
Labs	CBC: moderate **leukopenia**.
Imaging	CXR: within normal limits.
Treatment	Discontinue chloroquine or change to mefloquine as prophylaxis.
Discussion	Chloroquine, a 4-aminoquinoline (acts by blocking DNA and RNA synthesis), is still one of the most widely used drugs for the prophylaxis and treatment of malaria, although resistant strains are becoming increasingly common. Its side effects include headache, dizziness, defects in lens accommodation with frontal heaviness, epigastralgia, diarrhea, and itching (primarily in dark-skinned people). It is also used to treat amebiasis, rheumatoid arthritis, and lupus erythematosus. When taken for long periods, it produces retinal edema with macular hyperpigmentation and chloroquine deposits with visual field defects as well as semicircular corneal opacities.

CHLOROQUINE TOXICITY

ID/CC	A 25-year-old male presents with **spiking fevers, malaise, left-sided chest pain**, and **cough**.
HPI	His symptoms started two weeks ago and have progressively worsened despite a full course of oral antibiotics. He also reports a history of prior **IV drug abuse**.
PE	VS: **fever** (39.2°C); **tachycardia** (HR 105); **tachypnea**. PE: "amphoric" breath sounds heard over left lower lobe; S1 and S2 normally heard without murmurs, gallops or rubs.
Labs	CBC: **leukocytosis, predominantly neutrophilic**. Blood cultures negative; Induced sputum cultures grew **methicillin-resistant Staphylococcus aureus**.
Imaging	XR, chest: 2- by 3-cm cavity in left lower lobe of lung with air-fluid level. CT, chest: confirmed a left lower lobe **lung abscess**.
Treatment	Intravenous **vancomycin** therapy; add an **aminoglycoside** for synergistic bactericidal effect.
Discussion	**Antibiotic resistance** is continuing to increase in both the hospital (nosocomial infections) and the community. Major resistant nosocomial organisms include **S. aureus, vancomycin-resistant enterococcus (VRE),** *Klebsiella, Enterobacter, Escherichia coli, Pseudomonas,* and *Acinetobacter.* Multidrug-resistant bacteria causing community-acquired infections include **pneumococcus, gonococcus,** *Mycobacterium tuberculosis,* **group A streptococci, and E. coli.** Methicillin-resistant *S. aureus* (MRSA) is becoming widespread in a number of communities and is more commonly seen in **IV drug abusers, patients with recent hospitalizations**, and **residents in chronic care facilities**. Antibiotic resistance arises from numerous factors, including **colonization in hospital patients** and **frequent antibiotic use/abuse in the community**.

ID/CC A 21-year-old college baseball player restarted his training 3 days ago, running 1,600 meters a day in preparation for the upcoming state tournament; yesterday he hit a home run and started off to first base when he suddenly fell to the ground and **could not walk** due to **acute pain** in the **Achilles tendon**.

HPI He had spent 4 weeks in the hospital recovering from perforated appendicitis with peritonitis, where he received **IV ciprofloxacin** for 2 weeks due to a surgical wound infection with *Pseudomonas aeruginosa* that was resistant to all other antibiotics.

PE Surgical wound completely healed with no evidence of infection or postincisional hernia; Penrose drain orifice within normal limits; **inability to plantarflex left foot; Achilles tendon completely severed**.

Labs CBC: no leukocytosis; no anemia. SMA-7 normal. UA: normal.

Imaging CXR/KUB: within normal limits.

Micro Pathology Achilles tendon shows inflammatory neutrophilic infiltrate with areas of hemorrhage and necrosis.

Treatment Surgical repair.

Discussion Fluoroquinolones such as ciprofloxacin and norfloxacin are bactericidal antibiotics that are active against gram-negative rods, including *Pseudomonas*; they are also active against *Neisseria* and some gram-positive organisms. They act by **inhibiting DNA gyrase** (TOPOISOMERASE II). Side effects include **damage to cartilage** (contraindicated in pregnancy and small children), tendonitis, and tendon rupture; they also produce gastric upset and nausea and may cause superinfections.

FLUOROQUINOLONE SIDE EFFECTS

ID/CC	A 34-year-old woman presents with her family practitioner complaining of **hearing loss, vertigo**, and inability to walk properly due to **lack of balance**.
HPI	She is an otherwise healthy individual who underwent a left salpingectomy for pyosalpinx and was put on IV **gentamicin** for 10 days.
PE	Well hydrated, oriented, cooperative; gait is ataxic; abdomen shows well-healed, infraumbilical midline scar with no evidence of post-op hernia, infection, or hematoma.
Labs	**Elevated BUN** and **serum creatinine**; fractional excretion of sodium markedly increased ($> 1\%$). UA: **dark brown granular casts** with free renal tubular epithelial cells and epithelial cell casts. ECG: normal sinus rhythm; no conduction abnormalities or signs of ischemia.
Imaging	CXR: fails to disclose any lung infection or cardiac abnormality to account for the patient's symptoms.
Treatment	Supportive. Discontinuation of the aminoglycoside; resolution of acute episode may be delayed if patient remains hypovolemic, septic, or catabolic.
Discussion	Gentamicin is an aminoglycoside and thus shares the ototoxicity and nephrotoxicity of streptomycin, kanamycin, amikacin, and tobramycin. Ototoxicity is mainly cochlear and marked by ataxia and vertigo. Nephrotoxicity is minimized if care is taken to hydrate the patient and keep serum levels therapeutic. Transient elevations of BUN and creatinine are common.

ID/CC   A 23-year-old marathon runner visits his sports-medicine doctor complaining of unsightly, embarrassing **growth of his right breast** (GYNECOMASTIA) as well as **undue fatigue** after training and a slight yellowish hue in his eyes (JAUNDICE).

HPI   Three months ago, he was put on daily oral **ketoconazole** because he had been suffering from a severe, refractory tinea corporis infection.

PE   VS: bradycardia; **fever** (38.1°C). PE: slight jaundice in conjunctiva; no lymphadenopathy; no neck masses; cardiopulmonary exam normal; no hepatomegaly; examination of skin reveals tinea corporis covering intertriginous areas, buttocks, and scrotum.

Labs   **AST and ALT increased**; serum bilirubin level increased.

Imaging   US, liver: mildly enlarged liver.

Treatment   Discontinue drug; substitute treatment with alternative antifungal (e.g., terbinafine).

Discussion   Ketoconazole is an imidazole that inhibits fungal synthesis of ergosterol in membranes. It is used for blastomycosis, coccidioidomycosis, histoplasmosis, and candidiasis. Major side effects are **hepatic damage, gynecomastia, impotence** (due to inhibition of testosterone synthesis), inhibition of cytochrome P450, fever, and chills. When taken with antacids or H_2 receptor blockers, its absorption is decreased. It dramatically increases cyclosporine levels.

ID/CC A 21-year-old male comes to the health clinic because of the development of **fever**, marked **itching** all over his body, a **generalized rash** with **joint swelling**, and **difficulty breathing**.

HPI He just returned from a trip abroad, where he had developed a **purulent urethral discharge** (gonococcal urethritis) and went to a local doctor, who gave him "two shots on each side" preceded by two pills (procaine penicillin and probenecid).

PE VS: mild **hypotension**. PE: in acute distress; mild cyanosis and difficulty breathing; eyelids, lips, and tongue **edematous**; large **hives** on hands and chest.

Labs CBC: leukocytosis (12,000 with 60% neutrophils). Lytes: normal.

Imaging CXR: normal.

Treatment Subcutaneous epinephrine, oxygen, hydrocortisone, antihistamines. Maintain airway and provide assisted ventilation if necessary. Severe reactions may result in laryngeal obstruction, hypotension, and death.

Discussion Penicillins are antimicrobial drugs that block cell wall synthesis by inhibiting peptidoglycan cross-linking; they are bactericidal for gram-positive cocci and rods, gram-negative cocci, and spirochetes such as *Treponema pallidum*. Most adverse reactions to penicillin are allergic reactions that result when one of its metabolites acts as a hapten. Anaphylactic (TYPE I HYPERSENSITIVITY) reaction involves antigen reacting with IgE on presensitized mast cells and basophils; it is usually severe and immediate. Penicillin may also give rise to a **serum sickness** (TYPE III HYPERSENSITIVITY) reaction, an immune complex disorder with a lag period during which antibodies are formed. This results in fever, edema, malaise, arthralgias, and arthritis.

ID/CC   A 19-year-old military recruit comes to his medical officer complaining of **red urine** and **orange-colored staining of his T-shirt**; he also complains that every time he takes rifampin, he feels as if he has the flu (flulike response).

HPI   He underwent a routine physical exam and laboratory tests prior to joining the military camp and was started on **rifampin** at that time (meningococcus was found in nasopharyngeal secretions, indicating a meningococcal carrier state).

PE   VS: normal. PE: muscular male in no acute distress; no jaundice, hepatomegaly, spider angiomas, or parotid enlargement; nonpruritic maculopapular **rash** on chest and **petechial hemorrhages** on limbs.

Labs   **AST and ALT** moderately **increased**. UA: **proteinuria**. CBC: **thrombocytopenia**.

Imaging   CXR/KUB: normal.

Treatment   Switch to ceftriaxone or ciprofloxacin for eradication of meningococcal carrier state.

Discussion   Rifampin is an antituberculous drug that acts by inhibiting DNA-dependent RNA polymerase. One of its major drawbacks is the rapid development of resistance if used alone. Other side effects include **discoloration of urine and sweat** with a yellowish-orange hue, **hepatic damage, skin rash, thrombocytopenia, tubulointerstitial nephritis**, and increased metabolism of anticoagulants and HIV protease inhibitors.

ID/CC	A 9-year-old girl is seen in the ER for vomiting.
HPI	Two days prior to admission she developed fever, chills, headache, myalgias, generalized fatigue, and cough. She was taken by her parents to a pediatrician yesterday and given **oseltamivir (Tamiflu)** liquid suspension for the treatment of flu. After taking the first dose, she began to experience nausea that progressed to **vomiting**.
PE	VS: **fever** (39.0°C); **tachycardia** (HR 110). PE: normal.
Labs	CBC: leukocytosis.
Treatment	Symptomatic and supportive treatment; continue to administer Tamiflu and monitor for improvement in flu symptoms; discontinue use if vomiting persists despite use of antiemetics.
Discussion	Oseltamivir is used for the treatment of **influenza types A and B** in adults and children; it decreases the duration and severity of flu symptoms if taken within 24 to 48 hours after symptoms begin. Along with **zanamivir**, it comprises a class of antiviral drugs called **neuroaminidase inhibitors**, which block the release of progeny viruses from infected cells. The most common adverse effect of oseltamivir is **vomiting**, which generally occurs only once and improves with continued dosing. Other events reported include **abdominal pain, epistaxis**, and **conjunctivitis**. Zanamivir can worsen pulmonary symptoms by decreasing peak expiratory flow rates in patients with underlying asthma or COPD.

TAMIFLU (OSELTAMIVIR) THERAPY

ID/CC A 19-year-old **red-haired** female visits her dermatologist at a local clinic because of a **rash** that appeared after she spent the **sunny** weekend hiking without sun block protection.

HPI Two months ago, her dermatologist put her on low-dose **tetracycline** to prevent acne flare-ups.

PE VS: normal. PE: patient **blue-eyed** and **fair-skinned**; red, non-pruritic, **maculopapular rash** that blanches on pressure on "V" of the anterior neck, posterior neck, forearms, hands, and face, sparing rest of body (rash is on sun-exposed areas of body); chest, abdomen, and neurologic exams fail to disclose pathology.

Labs CBC/Lytes: normal. LFTs within normal limits. UA: mild **proteinuria**.

Treatment Sun protection, both mechanical and pharmacologic, while taking tetracycline.

Discussion Tetracyclines are bacteriostatic antibiotics that bind to the 30S ribosomal unit, blocking synthesis of protein by preventing attachment of aminoacyl-tRNA. If they are taken with alkaline foods such as milk and antacids, GI absorption is decreased. Tetracycline is used both therapeutically and prophylactically for chlamydial genitourinary infections, Lyme disease, tularemia, cholera, and acne. Other side effects include **brownish discoloration of the teeth in children** (contraindicated in pregnancy), **photosensitivity**, aminoaciduria, proteinuria, phosphaturia, acidosis, and glycosuria (a Fanconi-like syndrome associated with "expired" tetracycline).

ID/CC	An asymptomatic **HIV-positive** 29-year-old male visits his infectious-disease specialist for a routine checkup; after determining his **CD4 count (410)**, the physician decides to start him on oral **zidovudine** (AZT) at a dosage of 600 mg/day.
HPI	Two months later, he returns to the doctor's office feeling very **tired** (due to anemia); he has also had two URIs and yesterday started **bleeding from his gums** (due to thrombocytopenia).
PE	VS: slight tachycardia. PE: marked **pallor; disseminated petechiae** on arms and legs.
Labs	CBC: **decreased platelets** (THROMBOCYTOPENIA); **decreased WBCs** (NEUTROPENIA); **decreased RBCs** (ANEMIA).
Treatment	Discontinue AZT and **switch to zalcitabine**.
Discussion	AZT is used as an antiretroviral agent in symptomatic patients or in those with CD4 counts < 500. It is often combined with another nucleoside reverse transcriptase inhibitor such as ddI (an adenosine analog) or ddC (a cytosine analog). To prevent resistance, a protease inhibitor is also added to the regimen. Protease inhibitors block the proteinase that cleave the viral proteins needed to bud from the cell.

ID/CC	A 59-year-old female visits her family doctor complaining of **chronic fatigue**, **muscle weakness**, and **cramps**.
HPI	She has been receiving **furosemide** for the treatment of essential hypertension for more than 1 year.
PE	VS: **tachycardia**. PE: **dehydration**; somnolence; muscle weakness; deep tendon reflexes slow.
Labs	Elevated uric acid. Lytes: **decreased potassium and magnesium**. ECG: flattened T waves and prominent U waves (due to hypokalemia).
Treatment	Treatment consists of replacement of fluid and electrolyte losses. Monitor ECG for cardiac abnormalities.
Discussion	Significant dehydration and electrolyte imbalance may occur in loop diuretic overdose. These compounds **(furosemide, bumetanide, and ethacrynic acid)** are potent diuretics that inhibit the Na/K/2Cl transport system, which can result in **hypokalemic metabolic alkalosis**. Potassium replacement and correction of hypovolemia can reverse this toxicity. Additional adverse effects include **ototoxicity, hyperuricemia, allergic reactions** (except for ethacrynic acid which is not sulfa-derived) and **hypomagnesemia**.

ID/CC A 40-year-old woman who suffers from **chronic arthritis and headache,** for which she takes several types of painkillers containing **phenacetin,** says she had an episode of severe, colicky pain in the right lumbar region in the morning.

HPI She adds that the pain radiated to the groin, her **urine was bloody,** and she **passed a small piece of soft tissue,** after which the pain subsided. The patient has not consumed any fluids since this episode. She also has a history of **recurrent UTIs.**

PE VS: no fever; hypertension. PE: **anemia;** neither kidney palpable.

Labs CBC: normocytic, normochromic anemia. **Serum creatinine and BUN elevated.** UA: **gross hematuria;** sediment with no crystals. Tissue that patient passed measures about 4 mm and is **gray and necrotic;** no crystalline material demonstrated.

Imaging IVP: classic "ring sign" of papillary necrosis—**radiolucent, sloughed papilla surrounded by radiodense contrast material in calyx.** US, abdomen: bilaterally small kidneys. CT: presence of papillary necrosis.

Micro Pathology Papillary necrosis and tubulointerstitial inflammation on renal biopsy.

Treatment Total **cessation of analgesic use,** adequate hydration, and control of hypertension. Regular surveillance of urine cytology will detect uroepithelial tumors, which may arise after discontinuation of analgesic agent.

Discussion Renal papillary necrosis is seen in middle-age females with migraines or rheumatic diseases who take large amounts of analgesics. Usually there is a psychological component in the compulsion to take them.

ID/CC A 76-year-old female comes to her family doctor complaining of **constipation** and epigastric pain as well as **weakness** and painful **muscle cramps** (due to hypokalemia).

HPI She has a history of hypertension, for which she has been taking propranolol and **hydrochlorothiazide** for the past several months.

PE VS: mild hypertension (BP 145/90); no fever. PE: well hydrated; funduscopic exam shows hypertensive retinopathy grade II; no increase in JVP; no masses in neck; no carotid bruit; soft S3 heard; no hepatomegaly; no pitting edema of lower legs; **deep tendon reflexes hypoactive** (due to hypokalemia).

Labs Hyperglycemia; increased BUN. Lytes: **hypokalemia; hyponatremia. Hyperlipidemia; hyperuricemia; hypomagnesemia; hypercalcemia**. UA: proteinuria; high specific gravity. ABGs: **metabolic alkalosis**. ECG: S-T segment depression; broad, flat T waves; U waves (due to hypokalemia).

Treatment Potassium-rich foods (chickpeas, bananas, papaya, citrus fruits, prunes), potassium supplement, or switch to potassium-sparing diuretics such as spironolactone and triamterene.

Discussion Thiazides, the most commonly used diuretics (of which hydrochlorothiazide is the prototype), are sulfonamide derivatives that act by **inhibiting sodium chloride reabsorption primarily in the early distal tubule**. They are used mainly in congestive heart failure, edematous states, and hypertension (they have a mild vasodilating effect). The hyperuricemia induced by thiazide diuretics can also precipitate bouts of **gout**.

THIAZIDE SIDE EFFECTS

ID/CC A 48-year-old patient being treated for a large abscess in his lower back develops **oliguria, hematuria**, and an extensive **erythematous skin rash**.

HPI The patient has been treated according to culture and sensitivity of the pus from the abscess against *Staphylococcus aureus* with **methicillin**. He has no history of allergy to any medications.

PE VS: fever (38.2°C); mild tachycardia. PE: erythematous **skin rash**; rales auscultated over left lung base.

Labs **Increased serum creatinine** and **BUN**. CBC: eosinophilia. Blood culture sterile. UA: mild **proteinuria; sterile pyuria**; urinary sediment shows abundant eosinophils and no bacteria.

Imaging US, abdomen: normal kidneys.

Micro Pathology Renal biopsy shows evidence of **tubulointerstitial disease**; inflammatory infiltrate in interstitium consists of a large number of eosinophils in addition to neutrophils, lymphocytes, and plasma cells.

Treatment Alternative antibiotic therapy and supportive management; cessation of offending drug often reverses disease.

Discussion Drugs commonly associated with acute tubulointerstitial disease include **penicillin, ampicillin, thiazides, rifampin, methicillin**, and **cimetidine**. This type II hypersensitivity reaction is often reversed with cessation of offending drug; if it is not reversed, it may progress to renal failure.

ID/CC A 50-year-old male presents with **flushed skin, headaches, upset stomach, photophobia,** and **blue-tinted vision**.

HPI He has been diagnosed with **erectile dysfunction** in the past and is currently on **sildenafil** (Viagra). He has no history of **diabetes** or of **cardiovascular, prostate,** or **anxiety problems**. He also takes cimetidine regularly for acid reflux.

PE VS: **hypotension** (BP 90/50). PE: **plethoric** face; **nasal congestion**.

Labs CBC/Lytes: normal. LFTs normal. ECG: normal.

Treatment Adjust medications as necessary to prevent **cytochrome P450 interactions** with sildenafil. In this case, switch the patient from cimetidine to another H_2 receptor blocking agent with fewer interactions (such as ranitidine).

Discussion Sildenafil, which acts by inhibiting phosphodiesterase, enhances the effect of **nitric oxide**, an endogenous **vasodilator** that relaxes penile smooth muscle and allows blood to flow in, producing an erection. Side effects are dose-related. Sildenafil is **absolutely contraindicated** when **nitrates** are used for treatment of **angina** and should be used cautiously in patients taking **antihypertensive medications** or with preexisting cardiovascular disease. Reported deaths due to Sildenafil are typically **cardiovascular events** in **elderly men** (> 65 years of age). Sildenafil is metabolized by the liver via the **cytochrome P450** system and should be used cautiously in patients taking cimetidine, erythromycin, rifampin, and ketoconazole.

ID/CC A 28-year-old female is started on **amantadine prophylaxis**; she teaches at a school where there has been an **influenza** outbreak.

HPI One week later, she started feeling **dizzy** and having **problems walking normally** (ATAXIA). An ENT consult ruled out middle-ear causes of vertigo.

PE VS: **no fever**; remainder of vital signs normal. PE: **speech** somewhat **slurred; gait ataxic**; no focal neurologic signs.

Labs CBC/Lytes/UA: normal.

Imaging MR/CT: no intracranial pathology.

Treatment Discontinue amantadine. Amantadine is not effectively removed by dialysis because of its large volume of distribution.

Discussion Amantadine is an antiviral agent that blocks viral penetration and uncoating. It also causes the release of dopamine from intact nerve terminals (sometimes used for treatment of Parkinson's disease). It is used as **prophylaxis against influenza A**. Toxicity includes cerebellar problems such as **ataxic gait, slurred speech**, and **dizziness**. Elderly patients with renal insufficiency are more susceptible to toxicity.

ID/CC A 24-year-old female visits her physician because of **pain in her arm** after spending all day cleaning the basement of her house; x-rays taken as a routine procedure revealed a **linear fracture** of the right radius.

HPI She is an epileptic who has been treated for 3 years with **phenytoin**. She states that she has been suffering from increasing **leg weakness** and persistent **lower back pain**.

PE VS: normal. PE: **increase in size of gums** (GINGIVAL HYPERPLASIA); no neck masses; no lymphadenopathy; chest normal to auscultation; abdomen soft with no masses; no neurologic signs; **hirsutism** present; linear right radial fracture; **tenderness of lumbar vertebrae and pelvic rim**.

Labs **Megaloblastic anemia**; BUN and creatinine normal; **glucose mildly elevated; increased alkaline phosphatase**; decreased levels of vitamin D; **hypocalcemia; hypophosphatemia**.

Imaging XR: right radial fracture; **shortening of lumbar vertebrae; generalized osteopenia and Looser's lines** (MILKMAN'S FRACTURES; PATHOGNOMONIC).

Treatment Switch to other antiepileptics; vitamin D and calcium and folate supplements; treat fracture, physiotherapy.

Discussion Phenytoin and, to a lesser extent, other antiepileptic drugs such as phenobarbital and carbamazepine may cause **vitamin D deficiency** with consequent development of osteomalacia (in adults) and rickets (in children). Fractures with minor trauma may be a presenting sign, as may bone pain and proximal muscle weakness.

ANTICONVULSANT OSTEOMALACIA

ID/CC A 45-year-old **female** comes to her family physician for an evaluation of frequent URIs (due to neutropenia) and gum bleeding (due to thrombocytopenia). She also complains of **double vision** (DIPLOPIA), nausea, **sleepiness**, and **dry mouth** as well as difficulty walking.

HPI She has been suffering from recurrent, severe, sharp pain on the left side of her face that radiates to the corner of her eye and is triggered by mastication or cold exposure (TRIGEMINAL NEURALGIA). She has been taking **carbamazepine** for several months, during which time her attacks have been much less frequent.

PE VS: normal. PE: well hydrated, oriented, and in no acute distress; **ataxic gait**; funduscopic exam normal except for mild **mydriasis**.

Labs CBC: **decreased platelets; decreased neutrophil count.** Coagulation and bleeding time increased. LP: CSF normal. No evidence of multiple sclerosis on evoked-potential testing; **AST and ALT** moderately **increased**.

Imaging CT, brain: normal.

Treatment Switch to phenytoin. Consider alternative treatment options for trigeminal neuralgia.

Discussion Trigeminal neuralgia is sometimes seen in association with multiple sclerosis, primarily in younger patients. Carbamazepine is chemically similar to imipramine and has been used for trigeminal neuralgia as well as for the treatment of partial and tonic-clonic seizures.

ID/CC	A neonatologist is called upon to evaluate a newborn with multiple birth defects.
HPI	The mother is a 17-year-old runaway who is homeless, had no prenatal care, and continued her habit of **getting drunk** two to three times a week **throughout her pregnancy**.
PE	**Low birth weight; small head size** (MICROCEPHALY); **facial flattening** with **epicanthal folds**; small eyes (MICROPHTHALMOS); **cardiac murmur** (diagnosed as an atrial septal defect); positive Ortolani's sign on left hip and lack of complete hip abduction on that side; chest deformed (pectus excavatum).
Labs	CBC: mild anemia. Increased AST and ALT.
Imaging	CXR: cardiomegaly; pectus excavatum deformity. XR, hip: congenital dislocation of left hip.
Treatment	No specific treatment available; treat each malformation/disease accordingly
Discussion	**Alcohol is the leading cause of fetal malformations** in the United States. Fetal alcohol syndrome may cause myriad abnormalities, both skeletal and visceral, but usually involves a triad of features: (1) craniofacial dysmorphology, including mild to moderate **microcephaly** and **maxillary hypoplasia**; (2) prenatal and postnatal **growth retardation**; and (3) CNS abnormalities, including **mental retardation**, with IQs often in the range of 50 to 70. In addition, fetal alcohol exposure leads to an increased incidence of **cardiac malformations**, including **patent ductus arteriosus** and **septal defects**. Risk is dose related.

ID/CC A 23-year-old female is terrified after reportedly seeing grotesque monsters trying to kill her while she had her left dislocated shoulder reduced.

HPI She injured her shoulder while rock climbing in Colorado. The doctor was called upon to see her immediately after the accident. She did not suffer major injuries but had a dislocated shoulder and was not cooperative enough to tolerate the procedure (reduction) without medication, so he anesthetized her with **ketamine**, atropine, and diazepam.

Imaging X-rays at time of injury showed an anterior shoulder dislocation.

Treatment The **addition of diazepam** and atropine often diminishes the hallucinogenic effect of ketamine.

Discussion Ketamine is an arylcyclohexylamine that produces a **dissociative anesthesia**; the patient has open eyes, and muscle tone is preserved (with sufficient analgesia to do major surgery and total amnesia). Its major side effect is **vivid hallucinations**, sometimes terrifying, upon arousal, mostly in adults. It is widely used in developing countries, in rural areas where there is no available anesthesiologist, and in short pediatric procedures (abscess debridement, burn wounds, dressing changes, etc.) because of its relative safety and lack of life-threatening side effects (such as respiratory depression, which is common with other anesthetics). However, it also causes cardiac stimulation with increased blood pressure and tachycardia.

ID/CC   An 82-year-old male complains to his doctor about chronic **nausea** and vomiting, **loss of appetite**, and **altered taste perception** as well as **involuntary tremors, chewing, and grimacing movements** (DYSKINESIA).

HPI   The patient also states he has been having **palpitations** and **insomnia**. He suffers from Parkinson's disease and has been taking **levodopa** for a long time.

PE   VS: **tachycardia** (HR 115); **postural hypotension**. PE: patient thin; typical parkinsonian gait; masklike facies; pill-rolling tremor of hands; **choreiform movements** of head and hands; grimacing facial movements.

Labs   CBC/PBS: **Coombs' test positive**; no hemolytic anemia. ECG: **premature ventricular contractions** (cause of palpitations). Urine and saliva are brownish in color.

Treatment   Minimize side effects by taking drug with meals or in smaller doses. Often, administration of carbidopa diminishes side effects. Tolerance to emetic effect may also develop. Antiemetics may be given, but these may reduce antiparkinsonian effects.

Discussion   Dopamine cannot cross the blood-brain barrier; however, levodopa, a precursor of dopamine, does. When this drug is administered, it is usually given in combination with carbidopa, an inhibitor of the peripheral dopa decarboxylase (thus increasing the half-life and plasma levels of levodopa). Dyskinesias are a common side effect, as are GI symptoms (nausea and vomiting) and postural hypotension. Arrhythmias, anxiety, depression, insomnia, and confusion have also been reported. The dose of levodopa must be slowly decreased, since **abrupt cessation** may result in an **akinetic state**. Many patients eventually experience a decline in efficacy with levodopa/carbidopa. They may develop an "on-off" phenomenon in which they suddenly lose activity of the levodopa and are "frozen." Other patients experience a more gradual decline in which the levodopa effect lasts for shorter periods of time.

ID/CC	A 16-year-old female patient undergoes **surgery** to remove an inflamed appendix and has a rare anesthesia complication.
HPI	The father states that the patient's paternal uncle died of an anesthetic complication. The patient has had no prior surgery and received general anesthesia in the form of **halothane** and **succinylcholine**.
PE	VS: very high **fever** (39.8°C); **hypertension** (BP 150/95). PE: generalized **muscular rigidity** with difficulty breathing, anxiety, and marked sweating.
Labs	CBC: leukocytosis with neutrophilia. Lytes: **hyperkalemia**. ABGs: metabolic acidosis. Elevated CK.
Treatment	Immediate treatment to lower body temperature, control acidosis, and restore electrolyte balance is critical to survival. **IV dantrolene** relaxes skeletal muscle by inhibiting release of calcium from sarcoplasmic reticulum. This allows muscle to relax and limits hyperthermia from muscle hyperactivity.
Discussion	Malignant hyperthermia is a highly lethal, genetically determined **myopathy (autosomal-dominant** trait). It is triggered by inhalation anesthetics (more commonly halothane), particularly those coupled with succinylcholine. The syndrome includes **tachycardia, hypertension, acidosis, hyperkalemia**, and **muscle rigidity**, and it appears to be related to excess myoplasmic calcium.

ID/CC A 32-year-old male is brought by his wife to the family care center of the community because of increasing **tremors, slowing of movements** (BRADYKINESIA), and **postural instability**.

HPI The patient works as a **chemist** at a leading pharmaceutical research company in Northern California and has a long-standing history of **drug abuse requiring hospitalization**.

PE VS: normal. PE: flat facies; **resting tremor; cogwheel rigidity**; impaired capacity for voluntary motor activity; speech slow, as are voluntary movements.

Imaging CT, head: no apparent intracranial pathology.

Treatment No effective therapy currently exists for treatment of drug-induced Parkinson's syndrome aside from discontinuation of offending drug.

Discussion Several drugs may produce Parkinson-like symptoms, including haloperidol and phenothiazines, which block dopamine receptors, as well as reserpine and tetrabenazine, which deplete biogenic monoamines from their storage sites. In their attempts to produce "designer drugs" related to meperidine, "underground" chemists have also synthesized a compound, 1-methyl-4-phenyl-tetrahydrobiopteridine (MPTP). The toxicity of MPTP is produced by its oxidation to **MPP+** (a toxic compound), which selectively **destroys the dopaminergic neurons in the substantia nigra**.

ID/CC A 21-year-old male who emigrated to the United States 3 months ago visits a neighborhood medical clinic complaining of apprehension, tremors, **dizziness, inability to walk properly, and double vision** (DIPLOPIA).

HPI He is a newly diagnosed epileptic whose understanding of English is very poor, so when his doctor prescribed one tablet of **phenytoin** every 24 hours, he thought the doctor meant one tablet every 2 to 4 hours.

PE VS: hypotension; bradycardia. PE: bilateral nystagmus with sluggish pupils; patient is slightly lethargic; ataxic gait; dysarthria.

Labs CBC: megaloblastic anemia. Moderate increases in AST and ALT. ECG: sinus bradycardia.

Imaging CXR: normal. CT, head: no intracranial pathology seen.

Treatment Gastric lavage or hemodialysis if acute overdose. Stop treatment temporarily; then resume at proper dosage.

Discussion Overdose may be lethal owing to the ability of phenytoin to induce CNS, cardiac, and respiratory depression. Certain drugs, such as INH, cimetidine, and sulfonamides, can increase phenytoin levels by inhibiting the microsome enzymes that are responsible for the metabolism of phenytoin. The rate of hydroxylation of phenytoin also varies among individuals as a result of genetic differences.

ID/CC A 65-year-old female with long-standing **osteoarthritis** presents with **bilateral lower extremity swelling**.

HPI For the last 2 months, she has been taking **celecoxib** for relief of joint pain and inflammation.

PE VS: normal. PE: JVP normal; S1 and S2 auscultated normally without any murmurs, gallops, or rubs; **mild, bilateral pitting lower extremity edema**.

Labs CBC/Lytes: normal. LFTs normal. ECG: normal.

Treatment Monitor for worsening edema; provide temporary relief with diuretics; may need to switch to an alternative NSAID.

Discussion Celecoxib is a nonsteroidal anti-inflammatory drug (NSAID) used to treat **osteoarthritis** and adult **rheumatoid arthritis**. Recently, it has also been used to reduce the number of **colorectal polyps** in patients with **familial adenomatous polyposis (FAP)** and shows promise in treating GI cancers. Celecoxib works by inhibiting **cyclooxygenase-2 (COX-2)**, but unlike other NSAIDs, it does not inhibit COX-1. As a result, there is a **reduction in the incidence of upper GI ulcers** as compared to aspirin, ibuprofen, and naproxen, as well as less interference with blood platelets/clotting. Celecoxib is contraindicated in patients who are allergic to sulfa drugs or aspirin. It can also cause **liver damage** and/or **edema**. The **efficacy** of **thiazide diuretics, loop diuretics, and ACE inhibitors** is **diminished** by celecoxib.

COX-2 INHIBITORS

ID/CC An 18-year-old high-school dropout is brought to the ER because of marked **restlessness, euphoria, anxiety, tachycardia, paranoia**, and **agitation**.

HPI The patient is a known **drug abuser** with an otherwise unremarkable medical history.

PE VS: marked **hypertension** (BP 185/100); **tachycardia** (HR 165). PE: **diaphoresis; tremor**.

Labs Amphetamine levels are detectable in **urine** and gastric samples. UA: **occult hemoglobin** (due to **rhabdomyolysis** with **myoglobinuria**).

Treatment Treat agitation, seizures, and coma if they occur. Hypertension best treated with vasodilator such as nitroprusside. Propranolol used to prevent tachyarrhythmias.

Discussion A variety of amphetamines are used clinically, including methylphenidate (Ritalin) for attention deficit hyperactivity disorder (ADHD). However, many of these drugs are commonly abused as well. Such agents activate CNS via peripheral release of catecholamines, inhibition of reuptake mechanisms, or inhibition of monoamine oxidase enzymes. Excretion is dependent on urine pH, with optimal excretion occurring in acidified urine.

ID/CC	A 20-year-old medical student is brought to the emergency room because his roommate noticed that he had been **sleeping all day** and awakening from time to time with **nightmares**; the patient then stated that **he wanted to shoot himself** and began to look for a gun.
HPI	He had just finished end-of-year exams in all his subjects, for which he had studied late into the night and had taken **methylphenidate** daily for several weeks.
PE	VS: mild tachycardia. PE: well-oriented with respect to time, person, and place but very **lethargic** and complains of a severe **headache**; funduscopic exam normal; no increased JVP; no neck masses; lungs clear; heart sounds with no murmurs; abdomen soft and nontender with no masses; peristaltic sounds increased (patient complains of abdominal cramps when these are heard).
Labs	Routine lab exams fail to disclose abnormality; urine tox screen shows only trace amounts of amphetamine.
Imaging	CXR: no cardiopulmonary pathology apparent.
Treatment	Hospitalization due to risk of suicide, antidepressants, supportive treatment.
Discussion	Amphetamines are used recreationally for their ability to produce a sense of well-being and euphoria, with sympathetic stimulation. There are also some medical indications for their use, such as hyperactive child syndrome. Amphetamines may be abused orally or parenterally or may be smoked. **Withdrawal symptoms** include lethargy, **suicidal thoughts, profound depression**, intestinal colic, headache, sleepiness, and nightmares.

AMPHETAMINE WITHDRAWAL

ID/CC A 19-year-old **epileptic** student is brought by ambulance to the emergency room in a **coma** after being found on the floor of her apartment.

HPI She had been feeling depressed for several months and, according to her roommate, had just broken up with her boyfriend. She took a **whole bottle of her antiepileptic pills** at once **(phenobarbital)**.

PE She was brought to the ER **unconscious, hypotensive, hypothermic** (35°C), and **bradypneic**. PE: no response to verbal stimulation; reacts only to painful stimuli; **bullae** on lower legs; deep tendon **reflexes slow** (HYPOREFLEXIA).

Labs ABGs: pronounced **hypoxemia** and **respiratory acidosis. Blood alcohol level also increased.** ECG: sinus bradycardia.

Imaging CXR: no evidence of aspiration (a common complication of sedative overdose due to diminished gag reflex and altered consciousness).

Gross Pathology Globus pallidus necrosis with pulmonary and cerebral edema.

Treatment Airway maintenance; oxygen; assisted ventilation; gastric lavage; cathartics; alkalinization of urine; warming blankets; consider pressors, hemodialysis or hemoperfusion. **Flumazenil reverses benzodiazepine overdose but not barbiturate overdose**.

Discussion Barbiturates facilitate GABA action by increasing the duration of the chloride channel opening; they are used as antianxiety drugs, in sleep disorders, and in anesthesia. Barbiturates **induce the cytochrome P450 system** of liver microsomal enzymes, thereby affecting the metabolism of several drugs. In overdose, death may ensue due to severe **respiratory depression** or **aspiration pneumonia**.

ID/CC A 6-year-old-girl is brought to the pediatric emergency room because she accidentally consumed large quantities of her sister's **"Vivarin"** stimulant pills.

HPI The child, a healthy girl with no previous medical history, mistook the pills for candy, as they were in a non-child-proof container in the kitchen cabinet.

PE VS: **tachycardia** (HR 175); **hypotension** (BP 115/60). PE: **extreme restlessness, tremors**, and **nausea**.

Labs CBC/Lytes/UA: normal. SMA-7 normal.

Imaging CXR/KUB: within normal limits for age.

Treatment Monitor patient for ECG changes. Treat tachycardia and possible hypotension due to excess β_1 and β_2 stimulation with propranolol or esmolol.

Discussion Caffeine is widely used as an appetite and **sleep suppressant** and as a **diuretic**. It has a wide therapeutic index; however, serious toxicity may result from accidental ingestion of large quantities. Beta-blockers effectively reverse the cardiotoxic effects of excess catecholamine release and stimulation.

ID/CC A 14-year old boy is brought to the ER by his anxious mother for **mild somnolence, mild stupor**, and **mild motor dysfunction**. The patient initially answers negatively to questions about drug use.

HPI Upon further private questioning, he reveals that he had been "smoking a joint."

PE VS: tachycardia; mild tachypnea. PE: **conjunctiva red** and injected.

Labs UA: presence of **cannabinoids**.

Treatment There is no specific antidote for marijuana intoxication. Psychological disturbances can be treated with psychotherapy and adjunctive use of diazepam.

Discussion The primary psychoactive agent in marijuana is delta-9-tetrahydrocannabinol, which is released during pyrolysis (smoking) of *Cannabis sativa*. Acute cannabis intoxication usually consists of a **subjective perception of relaxation** and **mild euphoria** accompanied by **mild impairment in thinking, concentration, and perceptual and psychosocial functions**. Chronic abusers may lose interest in common socially desirable goals. **Therapeutic effects include treatment for glaucoma, prevention of emesis** associated with cancer chemotherapy, and **appetite stimulation** ("THE MUNCHIES").

ID/CC A 24-year-old female of Ashkenazi Jewish background complains to her family doctor of **repeated URIs** (due to neutropenia), increasing **fatigue, muscle aches, and headaches**.

HPI She had been showing flattening of affect, suspiciousness, a delusional mood, and auditory hallucinations that were diagnosed as **schizophrenia** 3 years ago. She has been receiving **clozapine** treatment because other antipsychotics were unsuccessful.

PE VS: **fever**; tachycardia (HR 165). PE: patient in obvious discomfort; **pallor** (due to anemia); conscious and oriented to person, place, and time; **petechiae** (due to thrombocytopenia) on chest and arms; cardiopulmonary, abdominal, and genital exams normal; no extrapyramidal signs.

Labs CBC: pancytopenia.

Imaging CXR: No signs of lung infection.

Treatment Discontinue clozapine and institute alternate pharmacotherapy.

Discussion Clozapine is used for the treatment of schizophrenia and psychotic disorders that are unresponsive to other therapy. It blocks D_1, D_2, and D_4 dopamine receptors as well as serotonin receptors. Because of its low affinity for D_2 receptors, clozapine causes few extrapyramidal symptoms. Agranulocytosis occurs in < 2% of patients, but all patients must receive weekly blood counts to monitor for this potentially lethal effect. Other side effects include seizures, sedation, and anticholinergic symptoms. Agranulocytosis usually reverses with discontinuation of clozapine.

CLOZAPINE TOXICITY

ID/CC   A 32-year-old stockbroker is brought to the ER after police find him **hiding in an alley**.

HPI   The patient had been at a **party** with several friends. He admits to indulging in cocaine from a new dealer for the past 6 hours.

PE   VS: **hypertension** (BP 180/95); **tachycardia** (HR 160). PE: **restless, malnourished**, and **disoriented**.

Treatment   Monitor vital signs and ECG for several hours. There are no specific antidotes for cocaine use. Propranolol may be used with a vasodilator for treatment of hypertension and tachyarrhythmias. Dialysis and hemoperfusion are not effective.

Discussion   Cocaine is a CNS stimulant and an inhibitor of neuronal catecholamine reuptake mechanisms; hence, its use results in a state of generalized sympathetic stimulation, with typical symptoms including **euphoria, anxiety, psychosis**, and **hyperactivity**. Severe **hypertension, ventricular tachycardia**, or **fibrillation** may also occur. **Angina pectoris** in a young, healthy person is suggestive of cocaine use. **Myocardial infarction** secondary to **coronary vasospasm** and thrombosis have been described as well.

ID/CC A 36-year-old male, an ENT doctor, tells his psychiatrist that he has been feeling terribly **depressed** and **anxious** over the last 3 weeks.

HPI The patient has been in good health, but he recently entered into a **drug rehabilitation program** to **wean** himself **off cocaine**.

PE VS: tachycardia; BP normal; no fever. PE: patient expresses concern over his increasing **lethargy, depression, hunger**, and **extreme cravings for stimulants** such as cocaine.

Labs Basic lab work and tox screen are all within normal limits. ECG: sinus tachycardia.

Treatment No definitive treatment exists to alleviate symptoms of cocaine withdrawal and associated cravings. Bromocriptine, a dopamine agonist that is used in Parkinson's disease, has been reported to diminish cocaine cravings.

Discussion Symptoms of cocaine withdrawal may be due to enhanced sensitivity of inhibitory receptors on dopaminergic neurons. In contrast to mild physiologic withdrawal signs and symptoms, cocaine produces marked psychological dependency and behavioral withdrawal symptoms.

ID/CC	A 35-year-old plastic **surgeon** is rushed to the hospital by his wife after he is found lying comatose in his bed with a couple of **syringes lying on the floor** and his sleeve rolled up.
HPI	His wife states that her husband had been having serious financial problems; she has suspected drug use in light of recent **personality and mood changes**.
PE	On admission to ER, patient had a tonic-clonic **seizure; respiratory depression**; bradycardia; stupor; **pupils very constricted** (PINPOINT PUPILS); cold skin; hypotension; marked hyporeflexia; hypoactive bowel sounds; **needle "train track" marks** (stigmata of multiple previous injections).
Labs	ABGs: hypoxemia; hypercapnia; respiratory acidosis. Urine tox screen positive for opioids.
Imaging	CXR: **noncardiogenic pulmonary edema** (edema without cardiomegaly).
Gross Pathology	Pulmonary congestion and edema; inflammatory neutrophilic infiltrate of arteries in brain and lung.
Micro Pathology	Brain cell swelling due to hypoxia.
Treatment	Establish a patent airway, assist ventilation, correct acid-base disorders, hypothermia, and hypotension. **Naloxone** as specific antagonist (naloxone may induce rapid opiate withdrawal), with follow-up in ICU.
Discussion	Heroin is a synthetic derivative of morphine that is abused as a recreational drug. Health professionals have a higher incidence of opioid abuse, generally abusing medical opioids. Heroin abuse is a complex social disease that is linked with violence, prostitution, crime, antisocial behavior, and premature death; it may result in fatal overdose, endocarditis, fungal infections, abscess formation, anaphylaxis, and HIV transmission. Death may result from aspiration of gastric contents or from apnea.

ID/CC A 26-year-old female who models for photography magazines is referred to the dermatologist by her family doctor because of **persistent acne** that has been unresponsive to the usual treatment.

HPI She also complains of **constant thirst**, dryness of the mouth, and **frequent urination**. She has been diagnosed with **bipolar affective disorder** with **manic** predominance and was recently started on **lithium therapy**.

PE Sensorium normal; oriented and cooperative; **mouth is dry**; no signs of present depression or mania; face shows presence of **severe cystic acne** on chin, forehead, and upper chest with **folliculitis**.

Labs CBC: **leukocytosis**. Pregnancy test negative. ECG: T-wave inversion.

Treatment Acne treatment with isotretinoin (teratogenic), chronic, low-dose tetracycline, benzoyl peroxide.

Discussion Lithium is the preferred treatment for the manic stage of bipolar affective disorder; however, its mechanism of action on mood stability is still unclear. One possibility revolves around lithium's effects on the IP$_3$ second-messenger system in the brain. The onset of action may take several days, and side effects may be very bothersome, such as persistent polyuria and polydipsia (ADH antagonism), weight gain, and severe acne. It is contraindicated in pregnancy due to its teratogenic effect.

ID/CC A 40-year-old male was brought into the ER by his sister, who reported that he had dropped by her apartment **acting "drunk"** and **agitated**.

HPI The patient was diagnosed as suffering from major depressive disorder 1 month ago and had been on phenelzine **(MAO inhibitor)** for 3 weeks. He was switched to paroxetine **(a selective serotonin reuptake inhibitor or SSRI)** last week.

PE VS: **fever** (39.0°C); **hypertension** (BP 150/100); **tachycardia** (HR 110); **tachypnea** (RR 30). PE: **disoriented; agitated, diaphoretic**; neurologic exam reveals **hyperreflexia, resting** hand **tremor**, and **rigid extremities**.

Labs ABGs: **metabolic acidosis**.

Treatment External cooling; supportive care; **IV benzodiazepines** for agitation and seizures; antihypertensives.

Discussion **Serotonin syndrome** is characterized by an excess of serotonin in the bloodstream. The combination most frequently leading to serotonin syndrome is a **monoamine oxidase (MAO) inhibitor** given with an **SSRI**. Other drugs that can precipitate serotonin syndrome in combination with an MAO inhibitor or an SSRI include **opioids (dextromethorphan, meperidine)** and street drugs such as **cocaine** and **LSD**. In severe cases, serotonin syndrome progresses to **seizures, disseminated intravascular coagulation (DIC), renal failure, coma**, and death. **Tyramine-containing foods** such as cheeses and beer in combination with an MAO inhibitor, can also cause a hypertensive crisis. Patients should **stop using an MAO inhibitor at least 14 days before starting SSRI** therapy.

ID/CC	A 43-year-old art consultant in an advertising agency is brought to the emergency room with **severe headache, palpitations, ringing in her ears,** and **sweating**; she had been **drinking** and dining at a French restaurant.
HPI	Over the past several months she had seen several physicians for a variety of complaints before finally being diagnosed with **hypochondriasis** and given medication for it **(tranylcypromine)**.
PE	VS: tachycardia; **hypertension** (BP 180/120); no fever. PE: **pupils dilated**; no papilledema; no signs of long-standing hypertensive retinopathy; no goiter (hyperthyroidism may lead to hypertensive crises).
Labs	CBC/Lytes: normal. LFTs normal; no vanillylmandelic acid in urine (seen in pheochromocytoma). UA: normal.
Imaging	CXR: normal.
Treatment	Gastric lavage; activated charcoal; treat hypertensive crisis with alpha-blockers to avoid producing hypotension; external cooling to manage hyperthermia. Avoid tyramine-containing foods.
Discussion	Monoamine oxidase (MAO) is an enzyme that degrades catecholamines. When inhibited, catecholamine and serotonin levels increase. MAO inhibitors such as **tranylcypromine**, and **phenelzine** are used to treat **anxiety, hypochondriasis,** and **atypical depressions. Tyramine** is a catecholamine food precursor (normally degraded by monamine oxidase) found in **fermented meats, cheeses, beer, and red wine.** When taken together, tyramine and MAO inhibitors rapidly elevate blood pressure with possible encephalopathy and stroke.

MAO INHIBITOR HYPERTENSIVE CRISIS

ID/CC	A 27-year-old female is brought to the emergency room by her mother because of a **high fever** and **muscle rigidity**.
HPI	The patient's mother reports that her daughter is being treated with **antipsychotics** for schizophrenia but is otherwise in good health.
PE	VS: **tachycardia** (HR 165); **hypotension** (BP 100/50); **fever**. PE: **confused** with an altered level of consciousness; pallor; **diaphoresis** (due to autonomic instability); marked rigidity of all muscle groups.
Labs	CBC: **leukocytosis. Increased CK** (indicates muscle damage). ABGs: metabolic **acidosis**.
Treatment	Treat muscle rigidity with **diazepam** and **initiate rapid cooling** to prevent brain damage (fever may reach dangerous levels). **Dantrolene, dopamine** agonists (bromocriptine). Respiratory support.
Discussion	Neuroleptic malignant syndrome is a life-threatening complication characterized by generalized rigidity and high fever that occur in certain patients with an idiosyncratic reaction to antipsychotics, such as haloperidol and trifluoperazine hydrochloride. The onset of symptoms is usually within a couple of weeks after the drug is started; diminished iron reserves and dehydration are predisposing factors.

NEUROLEPTIC MALIGNANT SYNDROME

ID/CC	A 48-year-old male complains to his doctor about increasing anxiety, **insomnia, irritability**, and **severe cravings** for cigarettes and food.
HPI	The patient, a two-pack-a-day smoker for 20 years, recently **quit smoking**. He claims that he is **no longer able to relax** and has been having problems with his wife and at work due to impulsiveness.
PE	VS: **tachycardia** (HR 155); **hypertension** (BP 165/110). PE: patient **anxious** and **sweating**.
Labs	CBC: increased hematocrit. Hypertriglyceridemia; hypercholesterolemia.
Imaging	CXR: signs of chronic bronchitis and emphysema.
Treatment	Gradually reducing the dose of nicotine either in **transdermal patches** or with **nicotine-containing gum** is helpful in weaning smokers from nicotine addiction. Group therapy, hypnosis, psychological consultation.
Discussion	Nicotine produces **serious addiction** and long-lasting cravings upon quitting. Nicotine produces euphoriant effects; however, tolerance develops rapidly. The psychological dependence of nicotine is very severe and a major impediment to quitting the tobacco habit. It is sometimes stronger than the physiologic dependence.

ID/CC A 32-year-old male, the lead drummer of a popular rock band, presents to the emergency room with **high fever, a running nose**, and **severe diarrhea** as well as abdominal pain.

HPI He is a chronic user of multiple drugs and had been a **heroin addict** for 2 years until two days ago, when he decided to quit.

PE VS: **tachycardia** (HR 165); **hypertension** (BP 160/90). PE: patient has **lacrimation and rhinorrhea** and is thin, **anxious**, malnourished, and **sweating** profusely; generalized **piloerection** ("GOOSEBUMPS"); abdomen shows tenderness to deep palpation, but no muscle rigidity or peritoneal signs.

Labs CBC/Lytes: normal.

Treatment Treat electrolyte abnormalities resulting from severe diarrhea. Monitor vital signs. Consider methadone substitution; clonidine.

Discussion Tolerance to opioids is a true cellular adaptive response on many levels, including Ca^{2+} flux, G-protein synthesis, and adenyl cyclase inhibition. Withdrawal effects consist of **rhinorrhea, yawning, piloerection, lacrimation, diarrhea, vomiting, anxiety**, and **hostility**. These effects begin within 6 hours of the last dose and may last 4 to 5 days. Cravings for opiates may last for many years.

ID/CC	A 52-year-old college professor with a history of **schizophrenia** presents with **tremor and rigidity**.
HPI	The patient is **diabetic** and a **smoker** and has been receiving **antipsychotic** therapy for **many years**.
PE	**Abnormal facial gestures**, including **lip smacking, jaw muscle spasms**, and jerky movements around mouth; Increased blinking frequency and difficulty with speech.
Labs	All labs normal.
Imaging	XR, skull: calcification of pineal gland.
Treatment	Decreasing dose or switching to atypical neuroleptics is first step. Benzodiazepine treatment can often improve GABAergic activity and therefore alleviate symptoms. Propranolol and calcium channel blockers may be of use.
Discussion	Tardive dyskinesia is a syndrome characterized by late-occurring abnormal **choreoathetoid movements**. It is often associated with antipsychotic drugs (e.g., dopamine blockers) and is estimated to affect about 30% of patients receiving treatment (males and females affected equally). Predisposing factors include older age, smoking, and diabetes. Advanced cases of tardive dyskinesia may be irreversible, so **early recognition of symptoms is critical**.

TARDIVE DYSKINESIA

ID/CC A 26-year-old female is brought to the ER by her boss after **fainting** at work. The day before she had complained of a **dry mouth** along with **constipation and urinary retention**.

HPI She had a major manic episode of hyperactivity and productivity at work 2 months ago as well as auditory hallucinations, for which she was diagnosed with a schizoaffective disorder and has been undergoing treatment with the antipsychotic drug **thioridazine**.

PE VS: **orthostatic hypotension; tachycardia** (HR 108). PE: acute **depression; dryness of mouth**; inability to accommodate normally (with resultant blurred vision); funduscopic exam shows **pigmentary retinopathy** and **dilated pupils**; abdomen slightly distended with diminished peristaltic movements.

Labs Increased prolactin levels; hyperglycemia. ECG: flattened T wave; appearance of U waves; Q-T segment prolongation.

Treatment Discontinue offending drug.

Discussion Antipsychotic drugs such as thioridazine and chlorpromazine manifest a number of adverse effects, making drug compliance difficult. Muscarinic blockade produces typical anticholinergic effects such as tachycardia, loss of accommodation, urinary retention, and constipation. Alpha blockade produces **orthostatic hypotension**. Other side effects include **extrapyramidal signs** (AKATHISIA, TARDIVE DYSKINESIA, AKINESIA, DYSTONIA, CONVULSIONS). Pigmentary retinopathy is restricted to thioridazine use.

ID/CC A 5-year-old male is rushed to the emergency department after his mother found him playing with her purse, where she carries her **antidepressants** (imipramine); she noticed that the boy had swallowed a handful of pills.

HPI The child complained of **dry mouth, blurred vision, and hot cheeks** (anticholinergic effect); he also complained of **palpitations** (due to arrhythmias).

PE VS: tachycardia with irregular rhythm; **fever** (anticholinergic inability to sweat); hypotension. PE: patient **confused**; pupils dilated (MYDRIASIS); **skin warm and red; diminished peristalsis** with no peritoneal signs.

Labs Lytes: normal. BUN and CPK normal. UA: **myoglobin** present. ECG: occasional premature ventricular contractions (PVCs) and **prolonged QRS** and **QT intervals**.

Imaging CXR: no pathology found.

Treatment Gastric lavage, activated charcoal, physostigmine in selected cases. Dialysis is not effective for TCA overdose because TCAs have a wide volume of distribution. Treat arrythmias.

Discussion Tricyclic antidepressants (imipramine, amitriptyline, doxepin) block the reuptake of norepinephrine and serotonin and are used for endogenous depression treatment. TCAs are commonly taken by suicidal patients and are a major cause of poisoning and death. Intoxication or overdose may produce **seizures** and **myoclonic jerking** (most common clinical presentation) with **rhabdomyolysis. Death may occur within a few hours**. Other side effects are anticholinergic (**sedation, coma, xerostomia**, and **diminished bowel sounds**).

TRICYCLIC ANTIDEPRESSANT OVERDOSE

ID/CC   A 5-year-old male becomes **cyanotic** and has a **cardiorespiratory arrest** in the ER.

HPI   The child, a known asthmatic, had come to the hospital by ambulance 15 minutes earlier with severe **wheezing, intercostal retractions, nasal flaring, and marked dyspnea**. He was given inhaled corticosteroids.

PE   Immediate CPR was given, the patient was intubated, and assisted ventilation was administered. The patient came out of the arrest but then returned to his preadmission state of wheezing and respiratory failure.

Labs   CBC: **leukocytosis** (16,000) with neutrophilia. ABGs: mixed respiratory and metabolic acidosis with hypoxemia and hypercapnia. **Peak expiratory flow rate** (PEFR) **markedly reduced** (indicates severe airway obstruction).

Imaging   CXR: left lower lobe infiltrate compatible with pneumonia.

Treatment   Metaproterenol by inhalation until bronchospasms stop. Treat infection, acid-base/electrolyte imbalance.

Discussion   In a severe case of asthma such as this, a preexisting infection is usually the precipitating event. Inhaled steroids have no place in the treatment of an acute attack, as is also the case with sodium cromolyn (cromolyn prevents the release of mast cell mediators, useful for prophylaxis). IV steroids may be given but may take several hours to take full effect (they block leukotriene synthesis by blocking synthesis of phospholipase A2). **Inhaled beta-agonists are the mainstay of acute, emergent therapy** (they activate adenyl cyclase and thereby increase cAMP, which relaxes bronchial smooth muscle). Adverse effects include arrhythmias, tachycardia, and tremors.

ID/CC	A 42-year-old female presents to her family doctor because of increasing concern over a **facial rash** for the last 2 months that cannot be concealed with cosmetics.
HPI	She has also noticed **joint pains** in the knees and sacral region as well as diarrhea. For the past 6 months, she has been treated with **procainamide** for a supraventricular arrhythmia.
PE	Hyperpigmented, brownish **butterfly rash** over the malar region. Left lung is hypoventilated, with dullness to percussion and decreased fremitus (PLEURAL EFFUSION); there is also a pericardial friction rub (due to pericarditis).
Labs	**Increased antinuclear antibody (ANA) titer**. Positive antihistone antibodies UA: **proteinuria** (> 0.5 mg/dL/day); presence of **cellular casts**. ECG: S-T, T-wave changes (suggestive of pericarditis).
Imaging	CXR: small left pleural effusion and enlargement of cardiac silhouette (due to pericardial effusion).
Treatment	Discontinue procainamide therapy and consider other class IA antiarrhythmics. Lupus-like symptoms typically resolve.
Discussion	Approximately **one-third of patients** on **long-term procainamide** treatment develop a **lupus-like syndrome**. ANA titer is elevated in nearly all patients receiving this drug, which can also induce **pericarditis, pleuritis**, and pulmonary disease. Other adverse effects include rash, **fever, diarrhea, hepatitis**, and **agranulocytosis**. SLE-like syndrome can also be produced by penicillamine, **hydralazine** and **isoniazid**.

DRUG-INDUCED LUPUS

ID/CC	A 30-year-old man is brought to the emergency room in a **stuporous state** with nausea, **protracted vomiting**, and malaise.
HPI	He had been overtreating himself with Tylenol (acetaminophen) with up to 30 pills a day to relieve the pain and discomfort associated with a whiplash neck injury he sustained approximately a week ago.
PE	VS: normal. PE: **icterus; asterixis**; patient **confused** and **dehydrated**; funduscopic exam normal.
Labs	Markedly **elevated serum transaminases; elevated serum bilirubin; prolonged PT**; mildly elevated serum creatinine and BUN; mild hypoglycemia. ABGs: **metabolic acidosis. Serum acetaminophen levels in toxic range.**
Imaging	CXR: within normal limits.
Micro Pathology	Liver biopsy reveals overt coagulative centrilobular necrosis; cells appear shrunken and pyknotic with marked presence of neutrophils.
Treatment	**N-acetylcysteine as a specific antidote** to replete hepatic glutathione levels; supportive management of fulminant hepatic and renal failure; consider liver transplant in severe cases.
Discussion	One of the products of cytochrome P-450 metabolism of acetaminophen is hepatotoxic. This reactive metabolite is normally detoxified by glutathione in the liver, but in large doses it may overwhelm the liver's capacity for detoxification. Renal damage may occur because of metabolism by the kidney. Encephalopathy, coma, and death may occur without treatment.

ID/CC   A 61-year-old male is admitted to the internal medicine ward for evaluation of **weight loss** and an **increase in abdominal girth**.

HPI   He is the father of an African student who is currently studying in the United States. His son brought him here from Central **Africa** for treatment of his disease.

PE   Thin, emaciated male; marked **jaundice**; abdomen markedly enlarged due to **ascitic fluid; hepatomegaly**; pitting **edema** in both lower legs.

Labs   CBC: anemia (Hb 6.3) (sometimes there may be polycythemia due to ectopic erythropoietin secretion). **Increased α-fetoprotein; hypoglycemia** (due to increased glycogen storage); AST and ALT elevated; alkaline phosphatase elevated.

Imaging   US/CT, abdomen: enlargement of liver with multiple nodularities involving the vena cava; enlargement of regional lymph nodes.

Micro Pathology   Liver biopsy confirms clinical diagnosis, showing fibrotic changes and glycogen accumulation with vacuolation and multinucleated giant cells; pleomorphic hepatocytes seen in a trabecular pattern (may also be adenoid or anaplastic) with malignant change (hepatocellular carcinoma).

Treatment   Palliative.

Discussion   **Hepatocellular carcinoma** is frequently seen in association with hepatitis B virus infections and with cirrhosis. There is a dramatic predisposition to this neoplasia in Africa and in parts of Asia; it is the most common visceral neoplasm in African men. Causative theories include the carcinogenic action of aflatoxins on genetically susceptible individuals. Aflatoxins are produced by the contamination of peanuts and improperly stored grains (staple food in many African countries) with the fungus *Aspergillus favus*.

AFLATOXIN CARCINOGENICITY

ID/CC A 47-year-old obese male who has been a heavy smoker for 20 years (with COPD) visits his family doctor complaining of malaise, lack of appetite (ANOREXIA), and persistent **pain in his shoulders and lower back** together with **dyspnea and dizziness**.

HPI He recently had a recurrence of gastroesophageal reflux disease, and nothing but his **aluminum gel** relieves it, so he has been taking large quantities of it in order to relieve his symptoms.

PE Obese and **lethargic**; heart sounds with no murmurs; lungs have a few scattered rales in both bases; **petechial hemorrhages** in legs and arms.

Labs CBC: mild **hemolytic anemia** (increased erythrocyte fragility); platelet count normal (but there are abnormalities in function-adhesion). **Phosphorus serum level low**; increased LDH.

Imaging XR: no sign of osteomalacia (acute phosphorus deficiency, not chronic).

Treatment Phosphorus supplements and/or switch to other antacids or H_2 receptor blockers.

Discussion Aluminum salts (HYDROXIDE) are used as antacids in many preparations. They commonly produce **constipation**, which is why most compounds add magnesium for its laxative properties to counteract the effects of aluminum. Another side effect of aluminum therapy is **impaired absorption of phosphorus in the GI tract**. With diminished available phosphate, the concentration of 2,3-diphosphoglycerate (2,3-DPG) decreases, leading to abnormal tissue oxygenation (malaise, dyspnea) and muscle weakness (including respiratory muscles). Hypophosphatemia, if persistent, may lead to osteomalacia.

ID/CC A 48-year-old factory worker is brought to the ER after a **chemical spill** because of **difficulty breathing** and **irritation of the eyes and throat**.

HPI He denies allergies, previous surgical operations, diabetes, high blood pressure, infectious diseases, trauma, blood transfusions, and hospitalizations, and he is not on any current medication.

PE VS: normal. PE: patient conscious, alert, oriented, and in no acute distress; **ammonia smell** emanating from clothes; **marked hyperemia** of ocular conjunctiva and upper respiratory passageways; throat mucosa and tongue **edematous** with mucosal **sloughing** on the left side; no laryngospasm; lungs clear to auscultation; abdomen is soft with no masses or peritoneal signs; no focal neurologic signs.

Labs CBC/Lytes: normal. US: normal.

Imaging CXR: no evidence of pneumomediastinum (seen with esophageal perforation with ammonia ingestion).

Treatment Treatment depends on route of exposure to ammonia gas. Observe patient for upper airway obstruction due to inhalation injuries. For eyes and skin, wash exposed regions with water or saline. There are no specific antidotes for this or other caustic burns.

Discussion Ammonia is used as a fertilizer, household chemical, and commercial cleaning agent. Ammonia gas is highly water soluble and produces its **corrosive effects** on contact with tissues such as the eyes and respiratory tract, producing severe laryngitis and tracheitis with possible laryngospasm.

AMMONIA OVERDOSE

ID/CC A 10-year-old boy living near a pigment-manufacturing industry presents with a **burning sensation** in a **glove-and-stocking distribution** together with severe **bilateral arm and leg weakness**.

HPI He also presents with **hyperpigmentation** and thickening of the skin over his palms and soles. The child is in the habit of **eating paint**.

PE Hyperkeratosis on palms and soles; peculiar **"raindrop" depigmentation; Aldrich-Mees lines** over nails; neurologic exam reveals decreased sensation, decreased motor strength, absent deep tendon reflexes, and wasting (SYMMETRIC POLYNEUROPATHY) in arms and legs.

Labs **Arsenic levels** elevated **in blood, urine, and hair**.

Treatment Penicillamine or orally administered succimer (DMSA).

Discussion Arsenic is used in a variety of settings, e.g., as pesticides, herbicides, and rat poison and in the metallurgic industry. The intoxication may be acute, with violent diarrhea, liver and renal necrosis, and shock potentially leading to death. In chronic exposure, the neurologic symptoms predominate over the gastrointestinal symptoms. The liver and kidney are also affected in chronic exposure.

ID/CC A 37-year-old male is brought to the ER by ambulance after collapsing while at work at a **metal-plating** factory.

HPI The factory routinely uses **cyanide**-containing compounds in its chemical plating process. A coworker reports that shortly before the patient collapsed, he complained of feeling **nauseated** and having a **headache**.

PE VS: tachycardia (HR 165); hypotension (BP 90/50). PE: patient is experiencing **agonal respiration**, is unresponsive to external stimuli, and exudes a bitter **almond odor**.

Labs Measured venous oxygen saturation elevated (due to markedly decreased oxygen uptake).

Treatment Treat all cyanide exposure as life-threatening. Give supplemental oxygen. Cyanide antidotes consist of amyl and sodium nitrates, which produce CN-scavenging compounds (especially methemoglobin). Sodium thiosulfate accelerates the conversion of cyanide to thiocyanate.

Discussion Cyanide, one of the most powerful poisons known, is a chemical asphyxiant that binds to cytochrome oxidase, blocking the use of oxygen and producing fulminant tissue hypoxia and death in seconds if inhaled or in minutes if ingested. It is used in the photographic, shoe polish, fumigation, and metal-plating industries. Free cyanide is metabolized to thiocyanate, which is less toxic and easily excreted in the urine. Exposure to cyanide gas can be rapidly fatal; however, toxicity due to ingestion of cyanide salts can be slowed with delayed absorption in the GI tract. Administer activated charcoal if accidental oral ingestion is suspected.

ID/CC A 25-year-old male with **HIV/AIDS** complains of severe **shooting pains** in both lower extremities.

HPI The patient is currently taking two **nucleoside reverse transcriptase inhibitors: didanosine (ddI)** and stavudine (d4T), as well as indinavir (a protease inhibitor).

PE VS: normal. PE: **thin, cachectic** appearance; no evidence of sensory or motor deficits on neurologic exam.

Labs CBC: leukopenia; elevated MCV (associated with taking reverse transcriptase inhibitors). LFTs mildly elevated.

Treatment Discontinue ddI and/or d4T and replace with **non-nucleoside reverse transcriptase inhibitor** such as nevirapine. Analgesics, narcotics, tricyclic antidepressants, gabapentin, or alternative therapies such as acupuncture may be effective in treating peripheral neuropathy.

Discussion Didanosine is a nucleoside reverse transcriptase inhibitor used in HAART (highly active anti-retroviral therapy) for HIV/AIDS. Its main side effects are **dose-related peripheral neuropathy**, diarrhea, abdominal pain, and **pancreatitis** (1% to 10% risk). Didanosine is also associated with **increased liver enzymes** and **hyperuricemia**. It decreases absorption of numerous antibiotics, including ketoconazole, tetracycline, and fluoroquinolones, and concurrent administration is not recommended.

ID/CC A 6-year-old boy is brought to the ER because of **slurred speech, lethargy** and **severe vomiting**. The patient was "helping" his father in the garage when he saw an **antifreeze** bottle and, out of curiosity, drank it.

HPI On arrival at the local pediatric emergency room, the boy started having tonic-clonic **seizures**.

PE VS: tachycardia (HR 108); no fever; **hypotension** (BP 80/40). PE: **hyperventilating** and experiencing **convulsions**.

Labs CBC: leukocytosis (13,000). **Ethylene glycol found in blood; metabolic acidosis with elevated** osmolar and **anion gap**. Lytes: hyponatremia; hyperkalemia. BUN and creatinine levels normal. ECG: **premature ventricular beats**.

Imaging CXR: no evidence of bronchoaspiration of ethylene glycol.

Treatment **Administer ethanol** to saturate alcohol dehydrogenase, which prevents metabolism of ethylene glycol to its toxic metabolites. Administer **pyridoxine, folate, and thiamine** (to attenuate the effects of toxic metabolites). Treat convulsions with diazepam and monitor vital signs. **Hemodialysis** can effectively remove ethylene glycol and correct acidosis and electrolyte abnormalities.

Discussion Ethylene glycol is the predominant component of antifreeze and may be used by alcoholics as an alcohol substitute. Because of its **sweet taste**, children and pets frequently ingest antifreeze. Its by-products may cause **metabolic acidosis, renal failure (due to intratubular deposition of oxalate crystals), and death**.

ETHYLENE GLYCOL INGESTION

ID/CC A 2-year-old male is brought to the emergency room by his mother after a bout of **vomiting**.

HPI The child has been seen by ER staff physicians in the past for **numerous episodes of vomiting and diarrhea**.

PE VS: **tachycardia** (HR 140); mild **hypotension** (BP 100/60). PE: **hyporeflexia; muscle weakness**, and tenderness.

Labs Lytes: serum **potassium low**. BUN, CPK, and creatinine normal. ECG: no arrhythmias or conduction disturbances.

Treatment Treat fluid and electrolyte imbalances. Monitor ECG for changes and possible **arrhythmias** (cause of death).

Discussion Ipecac syrup is an effective drug when induction of vomit is necessary due to ingestion of drugs and poisons, mainly in children. The safety margin is wide, but deaths have occurred when **fluid extract** of ipecac has been administered (much more concentrated than ipecac syrup). Chronic ipecac poisoning should be suspected in cases in which children are repeatedly brought in with symptoms such as these. Reports of such misuse in cases of "Munchausen's syndrome by proxy" have been recorded. Intoxication may result in cardiomyopathy and fatal arrhythmias (ipecac contains emetine).

ID/CC A 5-year-old male is brought to a medical clinic because of an episode of sudden, **vigorous vomiting** with no previous nausea (PROJECTILE VOMITING) (due to encephalopathy); his mother adds that the child has been **behaving strangely** and has been **irritable**.

HPI He also complains of **weakness in his hands and feet**. The boy lives in an **old house** that was recently renovated (old residential **paints and house dust** may contain toxic amounts of lead). He has had episodes of abdominal pain in the past.

PE Pallor; lethargy; **foot drop** (due to peripheral neuropathy); retinal stippling; lines in gums (LEAD LINES) (due to perivascular lead sulfide accumulation); **wasting of muscles of hand with motor weakness** (hand grip 50%).

Labs CBC: **hypochromic, microcytic anemia with basophilic stippling**. Hyperuricemia. UA: **increased urinary coproporphyrin and aminolevulinic acid. Blood lead** and **free erythrocyte protoporphyrin levels elevated**; glycosuria; **hypophosphatemia**.

Imaging XR, long bones: **broad bands** of **increased density** at metaphysis.

Gross Pathology Marked edema of brain; peripheral nerve segmental demyelinization.

Micro Pathology Acid-fast intranuclear inclusion bodies in renal tubular cells, hepatocytes, and osteoclasts; bone marrow biopsy shows **sideroblastic picture**.

Treatment Separation from source of exposure; chelation therapy with CaEDTA or dimercaprol (IM), or by DMSA (succimer) or penicillamine (oral).

Discussion Lead poisoning may be caused by gasoline, eating flaking wall paint (as occurs in pica), or using clay utensils with leaded glaze. Poisoning is more common in summer due to sun exposure with increased circulating porphyrins. Lead binds to disulfide groups, causing denaturation of enzymes, and inhibits ferrochelatase and δ-aminolevulinic acid dehydratase, thereby interfering with iron utilization in heme synthesis.

ID/CC   A 28-year-old male, a professor of chemistry at the local high school, comes to the emergency room complaining of acute **retrosternal and epigastric pain** and frequent **vomiting** of blood-tinged material.

HPI   He admits to a **suicide attempt** through the ingestion of several teaspoons of **mercurium bichloride** (corrosive) from his chemistry lab. On arrival at the ER he had a **bloody, diarrheic** bowel movement.

PE   VS: **hypotension**; tachycardia. PE: pallor; skin cold and clammy; tongue whitish; patient is confused, **oliguric, and dyspneic**; moderate abdominal tenderness; **grayish discoloration of buccal mucosa**.

Labs   **Elevated serum creatinine and BUN**. UA: presence of tubular casts. Fractional excretion of sodium markedly increased; serum hemoglobin levels markedly elevated.

Gross Pathology   Acute tubular necrosis; acute irritative colitis with mucosal necrosis with sloughing and hemorrhage.

Treatment   Chelation therapy with dimercaprol and succimer (DMSA); supportive management of acute tubular necrosis.

Discussion   Mercury, in its multiple forms, is toxic to human beings. Organic mercury is the most toxic. Acute toxicity is exemplified by this case. Chronic mercury exposure produces **proteinuria, stomatitis**, and **CNS signs**, mostly in children. These signs include insomnia, irritability, ataxia, nystagmus, and convulsions.

ID/CC	A 46-year-old **homeless alcoholic** is brought to the ER by two of his friends in a **confused, incoherent state**; he has been in the ER on many previous occasions.
HPI	He appears unkempt and, as usual, **smells heavily of alcohol**. He complains of nausea, vomiting, and abdominal pain, is very anxious, and constantly repeats that he **cannot see clearly**.
PE	VS: tachycardia; BP normal; **tachypnea** (respiratory compensation to severe acidosis). PE: patient confused as to time, person, and place; speech incoherent; no meningeal or peritoneal signs; no focal neurologic deficit; **marked photophobia** when eye reflex is elicited; papilledema.
Labs	CBC/Lytes: normal. Amylase normal (methanol may produce an acute pancreatitis). LFTs: slightly altered (due to chronic alcoholic liver disease). LP: CSF normal. ABGs: **pH 7.2** (ACIDOSIS). **Anion gap increased; serum osmolarity elevated** (due to osmotically active methanol). ECG: normal.
Imaging	CXR: normal. CT, brain: normal.
Micro Pathology	Retinal edema with degeneration of ganglion cells; optic nerve atrophy after acute event has subsided.
Treatment	IV ethanol (ethanol competes with methanol for alcohol dehydrogenase, having a much greater affinity for the enzyme). Dialysis, folinic acid.
Discussion	Methyl alcohol (METHANOL) is degraded by dehydrogenase to formaldehyde and formic acid, both of which are toxic compounds that cause a high-anion-gap metabolic acidosis together with ocular lesions that may lead to blindness (due to **retinal and optic nerve atrophy**).

METHANOL POISONING

ID/CC   A 46-year-old girl scout guide presents to the emergency room of the local rural hospital with excessive **thirst**, weakness, protracted **vomiting, acute abdominal pain**, and **severe diarrhea**.

HPI   She has been in good health and states that during the camping trip she ate some **wild mushrooms** (about 6 hours ago) that she had hand-picked.

PE   VS: **tachycardia** (HR 165); **hypotension** (BP 85/40). PE: lethargy; disorientation; skin is cold and cyanotic; hyperactive bowel sounds on abdominal exam.

Labs   Liver transaminases and bilirubin elevated; PT increased; increased BUN and creatinine.

Treatment   Thioctic acid, hemodialysis, treat fluid and electrolyte losses aggressively. There are no proven antidotes for amatoxin poisoning. Liver may be damaged to such an extent that transplantation must be considered.

Discussion   There are many species of toxic mushrooms, with clinical pictures varying according to the specific poison involved. Those most commonly involved in the United States are *Amanita phalloides* (delayed intoxication) and *A. muscaria* (rapid toxicity). According to mushroom type, toxins may produce anticholinergic effects (mydriasis, tachycardia, blurred vision) or muscarinic effects (salivation, myosis, bradycardia). These types of mushrooms are often picked and eaten by **amateur foragers**. Toxins are highly stable and remain after cooking. They are absorbed by intestinal cells, and subsequent cell death and sloughing occur within 8 to 12 hours of ingestion. Severe hepatic and renal necrosis is also a common effect of the toxins found in *Amanita phalloides*.

ID/CC   A 33-year-old female with HIV/AIDS presents with a skin **rash**.

HPI   Two weeks ago the patient was placed on triple antiretroviral therapy with AZT, didanosine, and **nevirapine**. She denies fevers, nausea, muscle/joint soreness, headaches, or abdominal pain.

PE   VS: normal. PE: **nonpruritic, maculopapular, erythematous rash** diffusely spread across trunk, face, and extremities.

Labs   CBC: leukopenia. LFTs mildly elevated.

Treatment   **Temporarily discontinue or decrease nevirapine** dose and, if rash resolves, gradually **dose escalate** nevirapine to reduce risk of recurrence.

Discussion   **Nevirapine** is a **non-nucleoside reverse transcriptase inhibitor (NNRTI)** that directly inhibits HIV reverse transcriptase and is used as part of a 3- or 4-drug regimen to treat HIV. Other NNRTIs include **delavirdine** and **efavirenz**. Side effects of the drug include **rash, fever, nausea, headache**, and **elevations in liver enzymes. Stevens-Johnson syndrome** is a rare but life-threatening complication. Since nevirapine induces **cytochrome P450**, it interacts with many drugs, including cimetidine, fluconazole, ketoconazole, azithromycin, and rifampin; taking such drugs with nevirapine may increase the risk of a rash.

ID/CC	A 22-year-old white female who is a professional skier presents to the emergency room complaining of severe **malaise, dizziness**, jaundice, **very low urinary volumes**, and **fatigue**.
HPI	Following a recent skiing accident, in which she sprained her shoulder and knee, she took a total of 20 tablets of **diclofenac** over a 3-day period.
PE	VS: mild hypotension (BP 100/60); no fever. PE: severe dehydration; tenderness to palpation in epigastric area; **pitting ankle and palpebral edema**.
Labs	Lytes: **hyperkalemia**. Markedly **elevated BUN** and **serum creatinine**; urine osmolality increased; fractional excretion of sodium < 1%. UA: proteinuria.
Imaging	US, abdomen: normal-sized, normal-appearing kidneys.
Treatment	Volume replacement, metabolic correction, immediate withdrawal of NSAIDs, avoidance of all nephrotoxic medications.
Discussion	Use of NSAIDs, such as diclofenac can lead to acute renal failure via two mechanisms: (1) unopposed renal vasoconstriction by angiotensin II and norepinephrine; and (2) reduction in cardiac output caused by the associated rise in systemic vascular resistance (an effect that is opposite to the beneficial decrease in cardiac afterload induced by vasodilators). Thus, inhibition of prostaglandin synthesis by an NSAID can lead to **reversible renal ischemia, a decline in glomerular hydrostatic pressure** (the major driving force for glomerular filtration), and **acute renal failure**.

ID/CC A 28-year-old male comes to his family medicine clinic and complains of **increased bruising** over the past 3 days, as well as **bleeding from the gums** while brushing his teeth.

HPI The patient is an amateur weight lifter who recently tried to lift an excessive amount of weight but strained a muscle and has been **taking indomethacin** for pain.

PE VS: normal. PE: athletic male with significant **ecchymoses** on chest and legs bilaterally; blood pressure cuff leaves petechial lines on arms; blood sample site taken on his arrival for routine blood work has become a large ecchymosis.

Labs CBC/Lytes/UA: normal. LFTs: normal; **increased PT**.

Treatment Discontinue indomethacin. Vitamin K may be used in patients with an elevated PT.

Discussion NSAIDs are extensively metabolized and protein-bound. NSAIDs inhibit the enzyme cyclooxygenase, thereby inhibiting prostaglandin production, which in turn produces their antipyretic, anti-inflammatory, and analgesic effects. Aspirin in particular is an irreversible inhibitor, and therefore the production of new platelets (about 8 days) is required before its anticlotting effects can be reversed. Moderate doses of NSAIDs can bring out subclinical platelet defects in otherwise healthy individuals.

ID/CC A 30-year-old **farmer** is brought to the emergency room with **severe abdominal cramps** and **vomiting**.

HPI The patient is also **restless** and is **salivating profusely**. He has been working with a new pesticide for the past 3 months.

PE Patient is nearly **stuporous; cyanosis** with marked respiratory distress; **bilateral miotic pupils; marked salivation** and **lacrimation**; moderate dehydration; **hyperactive bowel sounds; fecal and urinary incontinence.**

Labs ABGs: marked **hypoxemia** with **hypercapnia**; uncompensated **respiratory acidosis. Prerenal azotemia** on RFTs. Lytes: **hyperkalemia.**

Imaging CXR is normal.

Treatment Specific therapy includes administration of **atropine** (to offset cholinergic effects) and **pralidoxime** (chemically restores acetylcholinesterase if administered early); supportive management for respiratory support and hemodialysis.

Discussion Organophosphates like parathion and carbamates are widely used as pesticides, and several nerve agents developed for chemical warfare are rapid-acting and potent organophosphates. All of these toxins **inhibit the enzyme acetylcholinesterase**, preventing the breakdown of acetylcholine at cholinergic synapses. Whereas the **organophosphates may cause irreversible inhibition of** the enzyme, **carbamates have a transient and reversible effect.**

ID/CC A 23-year-old female with **HIV/AIDS** presents to the infectious disease clinic for a regular follow-up.

HPI She began antiretroviral therapy with AZT, ddI, and **nelfinavir** 1 year ago.

PE VS: normal. PE: cachectic appearance with peripheral wasting and relative truncal sparing (**"lemon-on-stick"** appearance).

Labs CBC: normal. Lipid panel reveals **hypercholesterolemia and hypertriglyceridemia; LFTs elevated**.

Treatment **Diet, exercise**, and **lipid-lowering drugs** to reduce elevated cholesterol/triglyceride levels; monitor for onset of **diabetes**; consider **switching** or **discontinuing protease inhibitors** if necessary. **Human growth hormone** has shown limited benefit in the treatment of lipodystrophy.

Discussion **Nelfinavir, ritonavir, indinavir,** and **saquinavir** comprise a class of anti-HIV drugs called protease inhibitors. Protease inhibitors are most potent when used as part of a 3- or 4-drug combination in patients who have never previously taken anti-HIV therapies. Side effects include **diarrhea, nausea, rash, lipodystrophy,** and **elevation in liver enzymes. Lipodystrophy** refers to changes in body fat composition that are believed to be related to protease inhibitor use. Other aspects of lipodystrophy include **elevated triglyceride/cholesterol** levels and **hyperglycemia** that can lead to **insulin resistance** and **diabetes.**

ID/CC   A 5-year-old female is brought by her parents to the pediatric ER with **severe nausea, hematemesis**, and **abdominal pain**.

HPI   She had been playing "candy maker" in her parents' room, and an **open aspirin bottle** was found on the floor. The child is otherwise healthy.

PE   VS: **marked increase in respiratory frequency** (HYPERVENTILATION); **fever**; BP normal. PE: flushed face; lethargy; **disorientation; dehydration; generalized petechiae**; abdominal pain.

Labs   CBC: **thrombocytopenia. Elevated PT**. Lytes: normal. ABGs: respiratory alkalosis.

Imaging   CXR: within normal limits for age.

Treatment   Antacids may be used for gastrointestinal upset. Fluid losses should be replaced. Administer activated charcoal. Based on specific acid-base disorder, treat accordingly.

Discussion   Aspirin toxicity may be pronounced in doses that are only five times the therapeutic amount. Decreased prostaglandin production results in decreased pain, inflammation, and fever. Acute ingestion may affect the integrity of the gastric mucosa and alter blood flow, which are prostaglandin-dependent processes. Diagnosis often depends on patient history, since quantitative levels are often not available. Salicylates stimulate the breathing center, thereby producing hyperventilation and respiratory alkalosis. Salicylates produce a metabolic acidosis as well as ketosis, so at different times during an intoxication and depending on the dosage, there will be different, often mixed, acid-base disorders.

ID/CC   A newborn infant has **underdeveloped limbs** consisting of **short stumps without fingers or toes** (PHOCOMELIA).

HPI   Her mother took a drug for erythema nodosum leprosum, a severe complication of leprosy (HANSEN'S DISEASE) during the first trimester of an unexpected pregnancy; the drug was **thalidomide**.

PE   As described.

Discussion   Thalidomide is a well-known teratogen that was widely used during the first trimester of pregnancy as an agent for insomnia because of its quick sleep-inducing effect. It causes phocomelia, in which a child's limbs resemble the **flippers of a seal**, with failure of development of the long bones of the extremities. Several thousand children were born with this abnormality, making the medical community painfully aware of first-trimester teratogens. Thalidomide induces abortions and multiple other fetal abnormalities. Thalidomide, under highly regulated monitoring, is an effective treatment for complications of leprosy.

THALIDOMIDE EXPOSURE

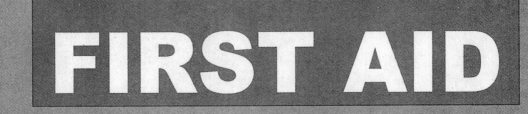
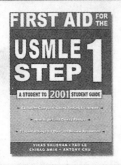
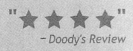
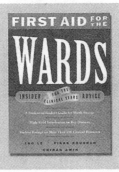
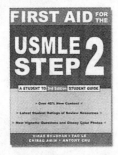
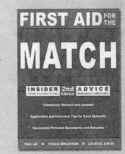
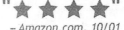
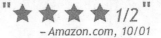